Moving Mama

Taking Care of Mother During her Final Years with Alzheimer's

By Rev. Dr. Anne Hays Egan

Edited by Pat D'Andrea

Copyright 2013, New Ventures Consulting
Registered with the US Copyright Office
All Rights Reserved

Second Edition, 2023

Table of Contents

Dedication v

Acknowledgments vi

Introduction 7

Chapter 1:   Difficult Discoveries.. 15

Chapter 2:   Trying to Make Sense of Things 25

Chapter 3:   The Will and The Government................................ 33

Chapter 4:   Protecting Her Finances 39

Chapter 5:   Standing Up to Others 49

Chapter 6:   A Change to Her Summer Visit 57

Chapter 7:   Hiring, Firing, and Blowing Smoke 67

Chapter 8:   Considering Options for Her Care........................... 77

Chapter 9:   Striking Out and Striking a Bargain 85

Chapter 10: Taking Care of Ourselves.. 97

Chapter 11: Packing and the Farewell Party 103

Chapter 12: Driving Down to Georgia 107

Chapter 13: Difficult Family Relationships 111

Chapter 14: Moving and Selling the Winston House 119

Chapter 15: When They Forget Who You Are 123

Chapter 16: Tough Choices and Taking Charge........................ 129

Chapter 17: Stories and Playacting... 135

Chapter 18: Getting Help Around the House 141

Chapter 19: The Magic of Music.. 145

Chapter 20: Friskies and Milk for Breakfast 149

Chapter 21: Health Problems, Hospital, and Rehab 155

Chapter 22: TSA Mishaps Mess Up Travel 161

Chapter 23: Afternoon Drives in the Bighorns 167

Chapter 24: Getting Her to Eat 171

Chapter 25: Dr. Whorton's RX for Skin Treatments 175

Chapter 26: Managing Sundowner's – Her Mother's Summer at Columbia 179

Chapter 27: Taking Time and Living in the Now 183

Chapter 28: Thanksgiving, My Last Visit with Mama 187

Chapter 29: Her Last Day – Debussy, Our Goodbyes and the 23rd Psalm 189

Resources for Caregiving 195

About The Author 203

DEDICATION

This book is dedicated to Mama; my aunts, Tula, and Sister; and my grandmother, Gram. They were all wonderful, strong Southern women who each were trailblazers in their own right. They left a wonderful legacy to those of us who now carry their stories.

- Hattie Hays Whorton, "Gram"   1882–1982
- Helen Margaret Whorton White, "Sister"   1904–1995
- Mary Carolyn Whorton Kinser, "Tula"   1911–2000
- Lorene Anne Whorton Egan, "Mama"   1917–2002

This is also dedicated to my brothers and sister-in-law, who were amazing caregivers, who made a positive difference in Mother's life, and our family.

- Thomas P. Egan and his wife, Ann Allison Egan
- John W. Egan

And it is dedicated to the friends and caregivers who helped ensure that Mama had a good quality of life. They were an important resource to Mother and all of us.

- Corinne
- Dotty
- Jolene
- Louise
- Mary and Baird
- Mary Pat at Agape and their caregivers

ACKNOWLEDGMENTS

I would like to thank my family, my brother Tom and sister-in-law Ann who cared for Mother in Louisville, and my brother John. They all were amazing and provided her with such exceptional care at the end of her life. Thanks also to Mama's caregivers and friends, who were so helpful: Mary and Baird, Louise and her friends from Parkway Presbyterian in Winston. Robin in Louisville. In Buffalo, WY, there were Corinne, Jolene, Dottie, Mary Pat and her staff, and friends at United Church of Buffalo, WY. Thanks to my Aunt Tula (deceased) who talked with us and with Mama so often; who provided calm counsel and support; and who was always there for her little sister.

To my cousins who read the book and provided such helpful feedback and suggestions, thank you Jenny, Carolyn, and Margaret.

A special thanks go to my friends who read the manuscript and provided wonderful suggestions: Betty, Catherine, Claire, Debbie, Jane Ann, Jerri, Michael, Vivian.

Thanks to my editor, Pat D'Andrea.

Introduction

My Mother, Lorene Anne Whorton Egan, was born September 28, 1917, and died December 17, 2002. She was the youngest of four children born to Hattie Hays Whorton (1882–1982) and Dr. William Walker Whorton (1877–1950).

We can say, like most families, that we had some family history that we loved to claim, as well as some rather bad behavior along the way, which we'd just as soon not. Although this has never been medically tested or proven, many of our family members believe that somewhere a number of generations back, some of our ancestors had "bad blood," as we say in the South.

Mother was a beautiful and brilliant child. She was an exceptionally smart and diligent student. Double-promoted in her early years, she graduated from high school at age fifteen, and entered the University of Alabama just before her 16th birthday, during the Great Depression. After graduating from college, she began a career teaching English at a high school in Birmingham, Alabama. Like most young single women of the time, she lived at home with her mother.

Mama was recruited by the American Red Cross to serve as a Club Director during World War II, which was one of the high points of her life. She and the group of young women recruited along with her traveled to the West Coast by train, and then went to Hawaii and Guam together. They spent weeks in training and formed close bonds. Many remained friends for the rest of their lives. Mother served in Guam and Tinian. She was there when the crew of the Enola Gay took off on their bombing run over Hiroshima, and was there when they returned. Like so many of what Brokaw called "The Great Generation," she said little about the difficult times. In fact, all she ever said to us about that night they bombed Hiroshima was they looked like they were in shock when they came back from Japan, and they were rushed off to a private debriefing.

Once or twice, she talked about how she and her staff would go onto the naval ships when they returned from battle and help the sailors write letters home. She did not speak about how many last letters they helped the young men write. Nor did she reflect about what the impact of hours spent with the dead and dying had on her own soul. In a letter she wrote to her mother sometime after the war, she mentioned that she could not imagine how difficult it must have been for families in Japan. However, those sorts of reflections didn't happen very often. Like Scarlett in ***Gone with the Wind***, she simply did what was needed. And, like her, she preferred to tell the more positive stories – like how, at the end of the war, at a celebration dinner, she met an officer who had just received a surrender sword from one of the islands. He gave the sword to her for her safekeeping that evening.

Mother had many stories and pictures about her time in the Red Cross during World War II. Some of my favorites include a photo with all of the Red Cross staff gathered together with their "house mother," Helen Merrill (of Merrill Lynch). She had kept lots of pictures of the club, people singing, and very few images that showed the dangers and horrors of war.

After the war, Mama returned to Alabama and was in charge of the Hospital Red Cross in Montgomery, where she met my father, who also worked for the Red Cross. Dad was given the task of teaching her how to drive. It must have been a very special Driver's Ed experience for them, because they dated and married.

After the war, many women were surprised to discover that much of their newfound freedom and occupational status quickly dissipated as the men returned to take back their jobs. In the Deep South at that time, many women were not expected to work after marriage. The Red Cross asked Mother to stay on as the Hospital Field Director after she married Dad, which was a tribute to her value to them. However, once she was pregnant with me, she had no choice but to retire into motherhood.

She was a full-time homemaker during the early and mid-1950s while they lived in Alabama. Then, in 1955, Dad received an assignment from the Red Cross to move to post-war France. He left before we did, which left Mama to pack us all up and stay in temporary barracks at Ft. Hamilton, NY, to await a ship to take us to France. I'm not sure how long we stayed in those temporary quarters awaiting orders and a transport ship, but I can remember being there, and it must have been a real hassle for Mama.

My father had found us a lovely old war-damaged chateau in Chambley, France, with rickety pipes. Pictures of us in front of the chateau show a beautiful front lawn with a circular drive. What you can't see in the picture were the problems with the plumbing and the electricity and the holes in the roof caused by bombing during the war. From the inside, you could see the sky through the holes. My brother, Tom, and I were forbidden to go up there. Of course, we had to check it out. In post-war France, we were lucky to have a roof over our heads, no matter how damaged.

The pipes in the house froze during the cold winter of 1956, while we were moving from Chambley to Metz. Gram came to spend a good bit of time with us in Europe. She took me to Paris with her many times on the train, and we went everywhere. She had permission to copy some of the artwork in the Louvre, and we spent a lot of time there. Paris remains one of my favorite cities to this day.

Mother drove me to kindergarten, which was part of a little one-room schoolhouse in Chambley. She made a home for us and managed our many trips throughout Europe. She introduced us to the history, art, and music of the countries where we lived and visited. I can remember standing in the late afternoon sunlight in Notre Dame, transfixed by the rose window. We spent one Christmas in Garmisch, following a terrifying trip through the Alps. My youngest brother, John, was born in the little military hospital in Chambley and has dual citizenship (US and France). He should make his native country proud, as he speaks the best French of all of us, and served as our French-speaking tour guide when all of us returned to Europe together many years later.

After our time in Europe, we settled in St. Petersburg, Florida. Mother managed the house and the children, and I can remember her walking us to the beach many times, taking a shortcut through the neighbor's yard. I remember visiting Dad's Red Cross office in the old Don Caesar hotel. It was quite interesting to discover on one of my consulting projects decades later that the hotel had been saved and renovated. It remains an area landmark, a gorgeous large pink art déco building. My father's office would have been somewhere in what is now air over the lobby entrance.

Following St. Petersburg, we moved to Pinehurst, North Carolina, and then to Montgomery, Alabama. Mama must have been thrilled to be back "home," and much closer to her mother. From this point on, wherever we lived, Mama and we three children spent each summer in Birmingham. Now that her children were all in school, Mother went back to work in the early 1960s. She taught music and had a staff position with the Girl Scouts. It was an extremely volatile time both in Montgomery and in our household. There were frequent arguments. Dad was drinking, and Mother was finding her voice.

Alabama was a very difficult place to live in the late 1950s and early 1960s. Montgomery celebrated its Civil War Centennial for most of 1961, and almost everyone I knew (white folks) dressed up in antebellum garb once a week to celebrate. Celebrate? The bus boycotts had just happened, and the Freedom Riders were coming soon. You could cut the fear with a knife. White violence was frightening and incomprehensible to me. To celebrate a mythic past during those violent days was like living in a danse macabre.

I remember my shock and dismay when the *Birmingham News* reported on the four girls who were bombed in the 16th Street Baptist Church in Birmingham in 1963. We were all there in Birmingham visiting Gram that summer. Adults whispered in attempts to keep their own fears away from their children. At thirteen, I felt I wasn't really a child anymore and wanted to know what the adults were saying. I remember overhearing Mama express sadness and concern over the senseless violence. That day, I spent a good deal of time by myself in Gram's backyard, just sitting and thinking. It was at that point that I began to realize that there was something fundamentally broken with the culture I had been taught to revere from the cradle on.

We moved to San Juan, Puerto Rico, in 1963, which made all the difference. Dad had been working quietly to get transferred out of Montgomery and its toxic influence. The move to San Juan was liberating for us children. Perhaps for Dad as well. I think it was probably more devastating for Mother than we realized. Dad's drinking increased, and Mother threatened to leave him, take the kids, and move back to Birmingham with her mother. She demanded that Dad go see Chaplain Diaz, who was the minister at the Protestant Chapel. He agreed to all of her demands, stopped drinking cold turkey, and focused on work and family. As time progressed, when he was not consumed with Red Cross disaster emergencies (like the Haitian Crisis where hundreds of people were airlifted from Haiti to Puerto Rico), he spent most evenings in the library or the woodworking shop until either closed for the day and he returned home.

Soon after she found her voice, Mother began to lose her moorings and have screaming fits. She would come completely unglued, running around the house, throwing things, and often hitting us. In public, we and our neighbors pretended not to notice. I babysat for most of the neighbors and was out of the house as much as possible. My middle brother mowed lawns and played golf. My youngest brother, John, was home and got the brunt of her craziness. That's what we called it. There were few mental health resources, and most people outside of New York and LA wouldn't be caught dead reaching out for professional help back then.

In spite of all of the discord and difficulty at home, we three children loved Puerto Rico. Living in a multi-racial culture was a new and delightful experience that shaped us forever. We loved going to a school with lots of other smart kids, and learning from teachers who loaded us up with challenges and homework. I attended Teen Bandstand at Ft. Brooke, and watched with amusement as my friend Bob Bird outfoxed the tourists who asked the 6'2" blond teen if he had seen Americans much, and he told them the long tale of his life as a poor Puerto Rican child, ending with 'Yeah, I lived in Chicago for ten years. It's OK.'

We traveled around the Caribbean. Mother signed John up for piano lessons and me up for violin lessons at the Conservatory of Music, and we attended the Casals Festivals each summer. Here, as in Europe and Montgomery, Mother was our family's director of culture and tourism. She was also an active volunteer in the church and community.

We moved back to the US and Louisville, Kentucky, in 1967 for my senior year in high school; not a propitious time. Mother began teaching piano in earnest during those years and spent most of the rest of her life as a piano teacher with many students and a full schedule. After the first year in Louisville, I went away to college. My relationship with her began to shift. Although I was not yet an adult in her eyes, and often didn't act like one, I was more than ready to try to strike out on my own. I was away for college and graduate school, and spent many of the summers at Brevard Music Camp. While I was in college, my father received his final transfer to run the Red Cross VA office in Winston-Salem, North Carolina.

They moved to a lovely place in what would be their last and long-term permanent home. For over thirty years, they lived in and loved Winston. By this time, they had built a nice asset base. Decades of deprivation and saving that had been drilled into them by early experiences in the Depression had now provided them with a very comfortable life. Their assets allowed them luxuries they had denied themselves in previous years. They enjoyed trips to the Outer Banks, and the Northeast (Dad's home area). They went to Europe and the British Isles.

My father became sick with lymphoma in the late 1970s. He managed a successful remission for six or seven years, then cancer recurred with flare-ups about every two years until 1992 when he died. He had the dubious honor of being Bowman Gray's longest-living lymphoma patient when he died, exhausted from life's battles. Tiny and jaundiced, he asked that we take good care of Mother. We think we did. Dad had taken good care of us. He had left the brokerage accounts in Mother's name with transfer on death arrangements to the three of us, which protected the assets from excessive taxation, and gave Mother all she needed for her final years.

When my father died, Mother discovered that she was exhausted from years of caregiving. She was thin and became sick with an ear infection soon after his death. In the years following, she continued teaching, and still had a large piano class. She was the President of Presbyterian Women at the church for some years and active in the local Music Teachers' Association. The few years after Dad's death were very full, and she was quite happy. What we did not realize was that after my father died, she began to show some very early problems with her memory.

By the mid-1990s, we could see that she was slipping.

Chapter 1: Difficult Discoveries

Perhaps the changes weren't that subtle. But then we weren't expecting them. After all, Mother was very smart – double-promoted and sent to college at the tender age of not-quite-sixteen. In addition to being exceptionally smart, Mama was well-organized, and always in charge. So, the possibility of her having Alzheimer's did not really hit us until it was obvious.

I think that's the case for many of us.

But there we were in the mid-1990s, facing a conundrum that both stumped and frightened us. My brother was examining Mama's bank statement when a $12,000 expense caught his eye. It was rather hard to miss, since the mortgage was paid off, and Mother had few expenses. Gradually, we pulled the story out of her. She explained that some very nice men had come by her house one day and told her they were roofers who were concerned about her roof. They explained they noticed some problems with her roof that needed to be addressed quickly before other problems developed and winter came.

We had to pull that story out of her a little bit at a time over many days and weeks. She was unwilling to talk much about it and was defensive. At some level, she must have had concerns about the huge expenditure. Perhaps she realized that she might have been duped and was ashamed. It was hard for her to share with us.

Finally, in bits and pieces, we got the gist of the situation. Being full of Southern hospitality, Mother chatted with them and allowed them to show her the areas where the roof was damaged. It seems as if, after not much more than a little conversation, Mother agreed to have them repair the roof. As she defended the expense, she explained that they were "very nice young men." She told us that she knew it was all right. "They had such nice manners, and even took me to the bank to get the funds." Indeed, they did take her to the bank, and to the cleaners!

The roof repair was minimal at best, and something that should have cost about a third of what she paid. For years, we had been hearing about schemes to defraud the elderly, and figured it couldn't happen to us because, after all, Mama was smart.

But Mama was also starting to lose some of that sharpness. She was also Southern, which means having good manners counted for a great deal. Many of these scammers seem to have a built-in radar for detecting the "mark's" weaknesses and zeroing right in for the hit.

We didn't realize it at the time, but manners and social skills would become increasingly important to her as her mind began to fail. Later on, they would help her to navigate the confusing world of dementia with a little bit more grace than would have otherwise been the case. We also didn't realize it, but we were all in some level of denial. After all, Mama was smart, we would think to ourselves.

After some initial defensiveness about the roofing job, she gradually realized that she had spent too much, and had placed herself in potential danger by relying so heavily on strangers. This was one of the first times that we noticed she was slipping.

Like many with early Alzheimer's, she was lucid most of the time. Until that point, the mental slips and moments of forgetfulness appeared infrequently and with little consequence. However, the roof repair illustrated just how vulnerable and isolated she was becoming. She was connecting less with others, and her circle was diminishing as she stayed home and alone most of the time.

It frightened us, and we began talking with one another more about the situation – and our fears.

We wondered if Mama was starting to get senile and discussed that fear in almost hushed tones. It was like "The Big C." As a culture, we've often stuttered over words like "Cancer." We often do the same with "Alzheimer's." It's like, if we say it, then it will happen. That's the big worry, isn't it?

As much as we didn't want to, we began looking more carefully at Mama. We researched Alzheimer's disease. We schooled ourselves in the signs and symptoms of dementia. There were times that I felt awful about doing that – like it was some sort of disloyalty to Mother to begin to classify her as someone who was becoming mentally impaired.

It's interesting, isn't it, that we often speak easily and openly about losing muscle tone and knee replacements. But losing mental muscle has such stigma still.

We discovered that the neighbors were doing most of the grocery shopping for Mother. She wasn't going to church as often as she had in previous years. Slowly, she was isolating herself, as is often the case as we grow older. We learned that those with dementia, or Alzheimer's, become isolated more quickly, and more completely.

As we worked with Mother over the coming year, we began to see other signs that she was slipping. We began to realize that she was suffering from dementia, probably Alzheimer's. It was awful to contemplate. When my brothers and I would talk, we would often ask each other if we were on target. "Is this really happening?" we would ask one another. "Is this what's going on?"

I was glad I had a background as a consultant in the areas of health and aging, because I knew where to start my research. But even so equipped, I found it difficult. There were days that I felt like Alice in Wonderland, down a rabbit hole and into another kind of reality. I read everything I could find from the Alzheimer's Association, which was a great resource. I had friends who recommended books, and I started to do internet research.

My brothers Tom and John were also researching options, such as ways to bring in more support to her at home. Sometimes when we talked, we felt like we were making progress. Sometimes we felt like we were stuck. We often doubted our own judgment. But as we continued to visit Mother and watch her, we found an increasing number of signs that she was, indeed, slipping.

Although Mother never liked to pay taxes, she always worked carefully and completed tax returns early. Like so many who survived the Great Depression of the 1930s, she didn't like to spend money or rely on accountants or other outside experts. She and Dad had developed good files, and a system for handling the multiple tax forms that included investment and capital gains income. How they could manage that, I still can't fathom. But they did. Mother and Dad hated to spend a dime more than absolutely necessary.

However, this year, Mother's tax forms were scattered all over her desk, along with files that were spilling their contents haphazardly from half-opened drawers, and some that were lying on the floor. She was organized to a fault. This mess of paper everywhere represented a significant change. The tax forms were just partially completed, with her name and address at the top, and big zeros at the bottom of the main 1040 form. As we talked with her about the taxes, she explained that she had been very busy, but that she would finish them "soon." She assured us that would be just fine, and that she did not need our help.

Like many of the WWII generation, she avoided discussing her personal finances with her children at all costs. Thankfully, she had forgotten that she'd provided us with Power of Attorney over her finances. My brother John was finally able to get her to sit down and talk with him. She explained that she didn't want to pay the government anything, and shouldn't have to pay the government because she was old, a widow, and near penniless.

Actually, she was right on just the first two counts.

John persevered once he saw she had started figuring from the bottom of the 1040 form, where she placed the large zeros. He was able to tactfully intervene to correct the forms and file a return more solidly based on reality. We were all very grateful to him, as it would have been difficult for us had she been indicted for tax fraud.

As we began looking around the house with a better grasp of reality, we discovered that she had posted dozens of reminder notes to herself. Mother always left herself reminders, but they were few and carefully written, usually close to the phone and her calendar. Now, the notes were posted all over the cabinet doors and countertops next to the phone. They included reminders to do basic things like talk with the neighbor about groceries, feed the cat, bill her piano students, and call the children. There were reminders on top of reminders. It was a patchwork quilt, and a disheartening discovery. Just to look at it was painful.

We also found out she was double and triple billing her piano students, often billing when a family's account was fully paid. Her group of piano students had been slowly dwindling from a high of about thirty students to less than a dozen at that point.

Within a few years, her base of students was to dwindle further to just three stalwarts who remained with her until her retirement party, which we gave her a few years later. Many of her former pupils came, and it was a delightful validation of her and her work. It was amazing that she was able to continue teaching for as long as she did. Her musical memory and piano playing were so much more lasting than her cognition.

Experts say that people who are musicians, or who play music frequently, are able to maintain their "musical memory" much longer than their regular memory when Alzheimer's hits. This was the case with Mother. She loved music. Playing the piano was one of her passions. She loved to teach, and she was very good. We supported her in her efforts to continue to teach until it became clear years later that teaching had become too difficult to manage. In time, we would discover how important music would be to Mother and to all of us as a way to connect when Alzheimer's had ravaged much of her brain. But I'm getting ahead of myself.

At that point in time, it appeared to us that, at some level, Mother knew that she was becoming forgetful. But she was fiercely independent, private, and committed to continuing with living as she had. She absolutely did not want to discuss anything remotely related to her memory loss. In fact, she denied having any problems whenever we brought up the issue.

She was also fiercely committed to maintaining her independence and living in her beloved house in Winston-Salem where she had lived with Dad for almost thirty years. The trouble was, she had become increasingly unable to maintain the house.

When we expressed concerns, Mother would make excuses, shift to another topic, or become intensely angry. Mama always lived a bit too close to the emotional edge, and we had learned many years ago to treat her with kid gloves, while watching for signs of an impending emotional storm. We realized that she was very prickly when it came to her living alone, her house, and her memory.

Often, when we mentioned concerns, she would say things like, "Are you trying to put your old mother away?" or "You think you know more than your mother?" or "Your dad would be so ashamed to see you treating me like this." With that kind of response, one does not usually continue with the same approach. We began to realize that the direct approach of mentioning our concerns was not very fruitful, and subjected us to barrages of anger from her.

We talked less with her about our concerns about her living alone and our worry about her managing her affairs, and more with one another when she was not present. We'd whisper our concerns when we were together at Mother's house. We talked frequently by phone, sometimes on three-way calls. We began to discuss options and strategies.

We worked to bring in more support for her, but, in time, she fired people we scheduled. We all agreed to visit Mother more often, and scheduled time each month that one of us would visit her and help her out with chores, housekeeping, and paperwork. That represented the first of many strategies we developed to help Mother (and us) deal with her Alzheimer's disease.

Reflection: Managing the Difficult Discoveries

Being willing to see these difficult changes can be one of the hardest and most heartbreaking of tasks. It's a challenge to face this issue early on. Nobody can prepare you for it. You may have an intellectual understanding of Alzheimer's disease from your experience with other older people, perhaps grandparents or other relatives. You may have had a close friend or spouse who went through this with their parents. It's possible that you know something about the disease from your professional work, as I did.

On one level, that knowledge and experience can be very helpful. On another level, it doesn't help at all. The knowledge and experience usually helps us later, after we have come to terms with the fact that our loved one has Alzheimer's and will be getting worse. It doesn't help us in the beginning to stare down our denial and our fears – and come to terms with the situation. We watch a parent start to forget things, cling to past skills, stumble over words, write little reminders, and we don't want to believe that can be happening. We don't want to see it for many reasons:

- *The possibility of a loved one living with Alzheimer's represents a devastating new reality, with them needing a lot of care as their cognition and strength diminish.*
- *It means a difficult and painful journey for them and for us.*
- *It suggests a great deal of future caregiving and a probable financial burden that can be extremely difficult.*
- *We don't want to start letting them go. A terrific description of that process can be found in* The 36-Hour Day.
- *We know upfront that it will be hard, though what many of us do experience as we go through it is sacred space and connections that we treasure.*

Check things out with friends and family. Read what you can. Start to develop your support system.

In the US, there are many web-based resources, like the Alzheimer's Association, National Council on Aging, as well as national caregiving groups. Other countries have similar resources. There is Alzheimer's Disease International and the Alzheimer's Association has an international website with links to specific countries.

In the US, there are important resources at the state level, which vary by state. Every state does have a department of aging, which is funded, in part, by the Older Americans Act. Local organizations like your local Senior Center can provide excellent information and resources, as well as much-needed emotional support. Many faith communities and local civic groups can also provide important support.

Chapter 2: Trying to Make Sense of Things

It is often difficult to spot early changes in memory and behavior because these changes are almost always slow and incremental. Like many people in the United States, the three of us were scattered across the country. Many grown children live at a distance from parents. If grown children live at a great distance, it's often the case that we see our aging parents a few times a year. Frequently, our parents lament not being able to see us more than they do. If we have children, the laments often increase in proportion to the number of grandchildren around.

It can take a while to build up a critical mass of information to convince ourselves and other family members that there is a problem. That was certainly the case with us. Until this critical mass is reached, most of us find ways to excuse behavior that doesn't fit, or is difficult to understand. Once family members realize that there is something wrong, we often move into high gear, trying to fix things. Sometimes we blame ourselves, asking "why didn't I see this sooner"?

In our middle years, most of us are busy with careers, caring for growing (or grown) children, and starting to worry about our aging parents. For the last decade or two, a growing number of middle-aged people are part of what's called the "Sandwich Generation," caring for both their children and their parents. We tend to feel guilty that we don't have enough time available to visit with them.

Most of us do the best we can with difficult circumstances that often pull at us from different directions. That stress can make dealing with a parent's aging issues that much more difficult. Know that you're doing the best that you can, and get support from friends and family as well as other and discuss options with the other members of your family and professionals that may be available.

In truth, it just takes time to realize a family member is having memory problems. That's probably a good thing. I wouldn't want someone jumping in to protect me from myself or institutionalize me at the first sign of my failing memory. I might be institutionalized by now if that were the case!

With Mother, we visited her more often. We took stock of the state of affairs when we arrived. Was the house clean, or in disarray? Had she been able to care for the cat? Did she have little notes to herself all over the place? Had she fired the housekeeper again? We would talk with friends and neighbors to see how they sensed she was doing.

Mama still had a few piano students left, and that was a helpful barometer. We observed how she taught. Her teaching skills remained excellent. She was attentive, resourceful, and wonderful with her students. However, with respect to billing, she was becoming increasingly confused and unable to handle scheduling and billing. We noticed that managing the scheduling and billing had been difficult for her for some time, and was now almost impossible for her. As a result, her base of students had dwindled to a dozen, and then a half dozen stalwarts.

So, what should we do? What can we do?

We continued to gather information and discuss the situation with one another. Each of us also talked with trusted friends whose opinions we valued. Some of our friends had already gone through caring for a frail elderly parent. My friend Nancy's mother was very ill and in need of care, and we would often share stories. Another friend and colleague had lost a mother years earlier, and talked with me about the grief that comes when facing a potentially long illness.

I remember when we were talking with Mother during the early stages of her Alzheimer's disease. A few years before our conversation about the roof, and before Dad died, the two of them had gone west to visit my brother John in Wyoming. Then, later on, after we became concerned about her forgetfulness, she mentioned something about our growing up in Wyoming.

We corrected her, but she kept to her story, and described in some detail where we had lived. It appeared that she had juxtaposed a mental picture of our house in Puerto Rico (where we had lived growing up) onto more recent memories she had from her trip to Wyoming. We could not convince her that she was wrong. In fact, she just became agitated and frustrated with us. We realized that, for us, once it was pretty clear there was a memory loss, the wisest course was to just go along with the statement or story, if possible.

When Mother continued to have problems with her memory, we decided one of us would go with her on her next visit to the doctor. At this stage, Mother was still lucid most of the time. She showed memory loss infrequently, and could often mask her difficulties. She had excellent social skills and was able to fall back on them to successfully hide her memory problems until later in the progression of the disease.

At her visit to the doctor, she was absolutely charming. She was able to win over the doctor, convincing him that she was fine and her children were unduly concerned and overly protective. The doctor deferred to her, and made some sort of inane comments. Mother had given an award-winning performance, and was definitely in rare form. As we got into the car to return home, she smiled and said something like: "Your old Mother is still on the ball, wouldn't you say?" What could we say? We (and the doctor) had been outsmarted, outfoxed, and outmaneuvered.

She knew it, and we knew it. She was so proud of herself and she crowed about her success.

It was at this stage that I looked for some resources to help me deal with the very tricky and challenging early-stage Alzheimer's that was affecting Mother. *The 36-Hour Day* was one of the first books I read, and I highly recommend it. There were a number of others I also found helpful, including Robert Butler's *How to Care for Aging Parents*. I had met Bob Butler years ago through my friendship with Maggie Kuhn, founder of Gray Panthers, and found him to be extremely insightful with an encyclopedic knowledge of the field.

During this time, I continued to be on the lookout to find friends and colleagues who had dealt with the issue. As people shared their experiences, it helped me to realize that the trajectory of the disease included many unsettling shifts, where people would sometimes appear to be their old selves, and other times mildly befuddled. Then there were those few times they seemed quite confused. As my brothers and friends and I shared, we realized the landscape was always shifting.

I came to understand that the ratio of confusion would shift over time, with her becoming increasingly confused and unable to cope. But, at the beginning, it was very unsettling to find Mother acting like her old self time and again, causing the three of us to wonder more than once if perhaps we weren't jumping to conclusions or being too hasty. Then, she would hit a difficult patch, and we would realize yet again that she was, indeed, declining.

I also realized early on that most adult children experience their own doubts as they confront the disease in a parent or other loved one. Self-doubt can be even more enervating when one is dealing with a spouse that is facing mental decline.

We can become angry. I know I was often angry to see Mother with diminished capacity. I was frustrated by the extra load we had started to carry. We loved Mama and were totally committed to giving her the kind of care that she gave her mother. We were committed to spending what was needed to do so. Even so, I was still filled with anger and grief and self-doubt on a regular basis.

Reflection: Making Sense of Things

It's important to gather information, discuss the situation, and ask for feedback from others who have been through similar challenges. Also, talk with other family members. Make notes about any changes you observe. Frequently, family members find that their loved one is a bit more forgetful and may repeat things.

People in the early stages of memory loss are more apt to forget recently learned information. But they can have good recall of earlier memories. Mother's problems with the roof repair, her tax return, billing students, and the increase in little notes to herself indicated a new pattern of forgetfulness. Taken alone, any one of those problems could have represented what happens when we are busy, overwhelmed, or distracted. However, taken together, they indicated the possibility of cognitive decline. The growing list of challenges showed a pattern over time for us, and will for you as well.

Early warning signs can also include changes in planning and problem-solving skills. People in the early stages of Alzheimer's often begin to show a level of poor judgment that is different from their norm. We saw a reduction in Mother's judgment with her quick decision to have the strangers who appeared to fix her roof. These scam roofers took her to the bank and to the cleaners!

In earlier years, Mother would have taken her time to make a decision, checking for multiple quotes, talking with a close friend or her sister, and looking into references. She would not have discussed this decision with her children, so that was nothing new. A number of experts indicate that financial skills are, unfortunately, some of the first to start slipping, so it is wise to be observant about changes in the way your loved one manages finances.

People showing early stages of memory loss may also have trouble finding the right words, and may start to stumble a bit in speaking, where this was never a problem before. People with an extensive vocabulary, like my mother, may be able to find other words (synonyms) and mask their difficulties longer than the average person. In fact, Mother's extensive vocabulary allowed her to mask her dementia with strangers for a long time.

Early in the trajectory of dementia, when stumped and unable to remember a word, she would simply substitute a synonym. In rare cases when that failed, she would raise her hands and say ... "well, you know." Synonyms seem to be an excellent preventive tool to address early-stage Alzheimer's. If we read a lot and engage in discussions about ideas, we build a diverse vocabulary replete with synonyms. That may be able to carry us for a while.

Most of us have periods where we doubt ourselves and our motives. We wish that we could do more and feel pulled between our own needs and the needs of our loved ones. That's a tough piece of real estate in which to reside. Most of us find ourselves in those places at least once, if not more often.

We were often on an emotional roller coaster, sometimes feeling confident and able to cope, and often feeling overwhelmed. Multiple times a day, my emotions could run the gamut from worried, upset, or angry to grateful, joyful, and hopeful. I began to understand that very little in my worldview, my work, or my relationships readied me to cope with and make sense of a senseless illness.

Get help where you can, from friends and family, community agencies, health and nutrition resources, spiritual networks and faith communities.

Most areas of the US have good local or regional resources to help adults who are caring for an elderly parent. Whenever possible, research and visit resources that may be available to help family members. I also recommend loading up on books, watching videos, and checking websites.

Other countries around the world have their own policies, care systems, funding mechanisms, and resource directories. There are helpful resources at Decade of Healthy Aging, AARP International, Arosa Care, Global Ageing, and the World Health Organization. These and other resources are included in the Resources Section at the end of the book.

Look for friends and family members who have lived through a similar experience and talk with them. If groups help you, look into a local or online support group.

Talk with family members who are sharing in some of the caregiving work. Research and analyze the local informal and formal caregiving options and supports that may be available. It's never too early to begin looking at what options are available for your loved one. It's always good to be equipped with information and a deeper understanding of options, based on research, discussions, and visits to facilities and supportive services.

Where possible, discuss together the pros and cons of your loved one staying where they live, moving in with a family member, or accessing assisted living or nursing home care. There are options for caregiving at home; however, many home care services are not covered by Medicare, though many are covered by Medicaid. Coverage levels and services available vary by state.

Discuss who among family and friends may be able to help out. Divide up tasks between family and friends who have offered to help out. If the tasks are shared and carefully managed, it can reduce the level of stress on the primary caregiver.

Develop strategies for ways to take care of yourself. Everything from little micro-breaks to days off and restorative activities that will feed your soul and recharge you.

Chapter 3: The Will and The Government

One of the frequent topics of conversation between my brothers and me had become 'What do we do with Mama?' We were at the point where we could no longer ignore her memory problems and her growing vulnerabilities. Dad had updated his will before he died, but we couldn't find it. After searching the house and talking over options many times, we all decided that we needed to get her to write a will – and soon.

We had just enough familiarity with the law to know that if Mother's mental state declined much more, it might be difficult to have the will declared valid if we were to run into any problems later. Since I was the next one scheduled to visit, my primary designated task was to get the will completed and signed.

All of the talk about wills also made me realize that the last will I had executed had also been years before, when I lived in Louisville, Kentucky. It was also time for me to update mine. I purchased one of those legal referral programs that allowed for a certain number of legal referrals to one of their participating lawyers during one's membership year.

I developed my draft and met with the lawyer. It was rather simple, and I had completed my will before going to visit Mama. Somehow, I felt that would give me some extra credibility and ammunition should I need it.

I needed it.

One afternoon, when Mama seemed to be alert and interested in talking, I mentioned that I had recently updated my will. "Oh, why did you need to do that? You're still young, and the lawyers just want to get your money," she said. "Oh, Mama. I wanted to make sure that everything I care about is taken care of." She didn't seem impressed. We talked for a bit, and somehow, I had an inspiration.

"You know, Mama. A good reason why I did my will is that I don't want the government to get any of my money." She looked at me and said with gravitas, "Well, I don't want the government to get my money either."

"Mother, if something were to happen to me. Say if I were hit by a bus, it wouldn't be right for the government to get my money."

She nodded and said again, "I don't want the government to get my money either."

"Not a penny," I said. She nodded and began to ask me more about how I had executed my will. I knew I had hit pay dirt.

I worked on a draft of her will, describing a simple division of assets equally between the three children, as I knew this is what she and Dad had planned for years, and was a cornerstone of the will that Dad had developed. She agreed. I also developed a Financial Limited Power of Attorney for my brother, John, with the other two of us as backups to him if needed. I could tell that she felt good. She mentioned a number of times being pleased that the government would not get her money.

The next day, I emailed files to the attorney and had the will professionally prepared. All that remained was to have the will and the limited power of attorney witnessed and notarized. We called her bank, and they set up a meeting for later that day.

As we drove over to the bank, I was both excited and worried. Quite frankly, I was very excited that we were accomplishing this important task, and rather proud of myself, if the truth be told. I was also worried about how Mother would behave. I knew we faced the possibility of some unanticipated difficulty. I could only hope that she would remember what we had done, and would agree to sign the documents in front of the bank officer and notary.

I hoped and prayed that she wouldn't suffer a memory lapse. These were becoming more frequent and unpredictable. It was becoming "the new normal."

I learned then an important lesson that was very helpful to us later as we continued to care for Mama. When she was in a public setting, she was much more agreeable. For years, even as her memory was clearly failing, when she was in a public setting, she found some strength and skill deep within her, and consistently rose to meet many an occasion that would have trumped a weaker person.

As we met with the bank officer, she was on her best behavior. Alert, friendly, and talkative, she was stunning. I marveled at her ability to meet some of her social challenges head-on.

My brothers and I talked about the will and power of attorney a number of times in the subsequent weeks. Sometimes we wondered if we hadn't pushed her a bit too much. We realized that many strategies ranked high on the sneakiness factor.

We had to settle for the murky middle ground of mixed motives. We wanted to protect her and us in the event that something happened to her. We knew it would be ridiculous for her to die without a will – intestate. Dad had made a will, which was somewhere. We believed we had honored his and her wishes to the best of our abilities. I knew that she didn't want the government to have any of her assets. I didn't want her assets, or mine, in time, so wasted.

Over the coming months, we would place a fair amount of attention on Mama's finances. They had scrimped and saved all of their lives, and had a sizeable nest egg. Dad had made sure to put all of the stocks and brokerage accounts in her name and ours, so that they would transfer upon her death to the three of us in equal proportions, with no tax liability. We wanted to make sure that her assets were preserved for her care, and for us, her children. And since she was losing her ability to manage them, we chose John to step in and help her make decisions. And then to make decisions for her.

When John visited, he would talk with her and help her update her bank balance. This was often difficult because she was unwilling to add any direct deposits as credits. Mother would think she was low on funds. John would carefully explain her income and expenses.

"John, I just don't have any money left."
"You're fine, Mama. You have money in your checking and savings accounts. And in stocks."
"But look at this. Right here," she'd say, pointing to an erroneous figure in her checking account register.
"Mama, your Social Security check goes from the government right to your bank account. It's there. See?"

He would show her the deposit record each time he visited, and she would reply, "But I never received the check, and I did not deposit it. So, if I didn't deposit it, then I can't add it to my bank balance." At least she underestimated her bank balance.

Gradually, John quit trying to explain this. We realized that, with early Alzheimer's, she didn't remember recent events very well. With this, we learned to be more strategic about what we discussed with her and at what level of detail.

Reflection: Planning Ahead and Managing Affairs

How do we even begin to tackle helping parents or other loved ones with their affairs? The first and most important thing is to have a plan. If you're lucky, your loved one may have already started planning for their final years, and can discuss their needs and priorities with you while they are still active. Today's older adults are more willing to discuss financial and personal issues with their children than was my mother's generation. You may be able to get a running start on caring for your elderly parents by working with them to find out how they want to handle their affairs as they become older and more frail. That's the ideal. It may or may not be possible in your case, but try to have these conversations if you can.

My mother, who was born in 1918, was very much an "old school parent," and did not discuss any of her personal business or finances with her children. That made it very difficult to build a plan with her. We had to start where we were able to start, which was when she began to show signs of slipping.

My brothers and I created a very simple plan, which we developed over time. The plan is a bit more organized in retrospect than it was as we moved through the process. Hindsight and time provide more clarity. While we were going through it, we put the pieces together to cobble whatever we thought was needed and would work.

Our simple plan:

I. *Plan for her care as she becomes frailer.*
  A. *Help her around the house.*
   1. *Visit her more often.*
   2. *Look to see what's happening, track what she needs and what she's able to do.*

3. Do chores and home repairs when visiting.
4. Try to bring in help where possible.
   B. Research options for her future living situation.
      1. Investigate assisted living or nursing home options.
      2. Put in place some additional support at home with housekeeping and the yard.
      3. Research and discuss home caregiving options.
II. Protect and manage her assets and her estate.
   A. Develop a new will.
      1. Write the new will and have it witnessed and notarized.
      2. Write and notarize a limited Financial Power of Attorney for John to handle her financial matters, including banking and brokerage accounts.
      3. Write and notarize a Healthcare Power of Attorney so that we could make decisions about her health should she become incapacitated.
   B. Manage her finances.
      1. Review her stock portfolio and ensure that the accounts are set up in her name jointly with the three children, with a Transfer on Death option.
      2. Review and oversee her taxes to make sure that she isn't filing incorrect information.
      3. Track her income and expenses, and manage her major expenses.

This was not nearly as neat and orderly as it looks now. It was messy and emerged gradually. We did develop the outline of the plan early on. We learned that, although all of the aspects of caregiving were challenging, some were harder than others. Each family is a little different. Having a plan will help outline the most important goals, identify who will do what, and serve as a roadmap for the journey.

Chapter 4: Protecting Her Finances

In retrospect, we realized that we had been very concerned about Mother's management of her finances for over a year before we were able to intervene. John had handled the tax situation brilliantly, and I was able to update her will and put into place a Financial Limited Power of Attorney so that John could begin to handle her brokerage and bank accounts with her.

It took a good bit of work to be able to manage her finances, and we learned what was most important as we went through the process.

The first clue that things were wrong was a change in her financial habits. Mother was one of those children of the Great Depression who managed frugally, and was always in control of her income and expenses. However, as Alzheimer's began to affect her memory, her skills began to slip.

Mother didn't have a lot of expenses. By the time she was in her seventies, the house was paid off, and she had few recurring monthly costs. However, she had sizeable bank and brokerage accounts that were at risk.

We realized that Mama was not tracking finances well when she began to double-bill her students and start her tax returns by putting a big Zero as the total. The roofing fiasco where she spent $12,000 on strangers in 1998 was a huge red flag for us. At this point, we had already begun to work with her on her will, managing her finances, and putting brokerage accounts in trust. When she spent $12,000 on the strangers dropping by to tell her she needed roof repairs, we moved into high gear. In the late 1990s, there were not nearly as many scams as there are today, but those that existed were scary.

We had all agreed that John was best suited to the financial oversight task for many reasons. John was the youngest and the peacemaker. My other brother and I trusted John to handle things in Mother's and our best interests.

All three of us supported this plan, and John agreed to keep us informed about her finances and to check with us about any large expenditures. He did that, and we tended to be in agreement about how her money was managed.

One other area where we were in agreement, which was actually rather amazing, was that we talked in general terms about how the money should be spent. We three agreed that whatever funds were needed to be spent for her care would be spent. We were lucky in that regard.

Mama had taken wonderful care of her mother, who lived to be almost 100 years old. That example became part of her gift to us, and part of our roadmap. We had grown up with the belief that one takes care of one's parents, no matter what. It's just what is done.

In addition, all three of us have worked in nonprofit, educational, and community organizations all our lives and have been steeped in those values. The fact that we agreed to spend what was needed for her care was a miracle, I think.

Mother and Dad had worked hard, scrimped and saved in order to build a good-sized nest egg, and we wanted our decisions to be aligned with her values. Our hope was to spend her money wisely to safeguard her and protect what would remain for us. For us, preserving her estate for us was a secondary, though important, emphasis. How that happened, I don't know.

John kept track of her income and expenses for years. He managed her money wisely and ensured that funds were well invested to preserve her principal. During Dad's final year, when he was very sick with cancer, he had made some unwise investment choices. He held onto his Pan Am stock when the airline was tanking, and that was when we knew that he was in very bad shape.

John started meeting with her broker and researching the stocks in her portfolio. He discovered that too much of her portfolio had been allocated into the broker's own "house stocks," which were basically garbage. Later, the federal government passed a law against this kind of in-house brokerage self-dealing. But before that, it was a bit wilder.

Ron, her broker, was a "good old Southern boy" who had gone to Clemson, pledged a good fraternity, and probably got his job through his family or fraternity brothers. He was not very bright. But he was very social and visited Mother on a regular basis. She liked him. He was a nice young man.

Once John started managing Mother's funds, he became concerned about this nice young man. John had filed the Financial Power of Attorney with Ron, and had talked with him about Mother's portfolio, and soon afterward, Ron's visits to Mother became more frequent. Not exactly coincidence.

Although Mama thought Ron was charming, we couldn't stand him. We knew that he had been churning her portfolio to benefit the brokerage firm, rather than investing in support of her goals in ways that preserved her assets. He was handsome, not terribly quick upstairs, slow, slick, and very successful at manipulating her.

After talking together by phone, we hatched a plan. We were all going to be at Mother's during the summer, and our plans allowed us to schedule a few days where our visits would overlap. We decided we would schedule an appointment with Ron. All of us.

John analyzed the portfolio. The three of us looked at other stock and mutual fund performance levels for comparisons. We also talked with Mama's sister Tula and our cousin Carolyn, who was helping Tula with her investments. Tula's portfolio had been managed much more effectively, and it helped to have another "take" on things. Tom and I developed some strategies for the meeting.

On the appointed day, the three of us descended on Ron's office. Although John had talked with Ron often by phone and met with him a few times, Tom and I didn't know Ron very well, but had met him occasionally over the years.

I was the most Southern of the three children, being the oldest and a girl. Having gone to Converse College, I still dressed and acted like a Converse girl. In my day, that meant a certain panache that came with matching clothes, the right jewelry, accessories, and shoes. It's a cross I still bear.

My brother Tom was and is, a big man with a very intimidating presence. John is both friendly and intellectually intimidating. Hell, we all three can be intellectually intimidating when we want to be. For this meeting, we wanted to be as intimidating as possible.

My role was to start the conversation. So, I greeted Ron in that superficial way that Southern near-strangers of a certain age engage in. Once we had him chatting away, John began to ask questions. Very pointed questions. He went over Mother's portfolio and identified those stocks that had not performed well, zeroing in on the in-house garbage funds.

Meanwhile, looking stern, Tom pulled his chair much closer to the broker's desk, and leaned forward, attentively. Ron began to flutter and stammer like a schoolgirl. He was clearly unprepared for the level of analysis we had conducted and the questions we asked. Ron was not gifted with a great deal of brainpower. He was unprepared, and didn't have good answers. As the conversation continued, he realized that he was in hot water and in danger of losing a preferred customer account.

The conversation ended with John informing Ron that he was in charge of Mother's account, and that all instructions concerning Mother's investments were to come from him. John provided Ron with a list of changes that were to take effect. He let Ron know that he would be managing the account closely, in frequent contact, and would pull the account if Ron did not handle things more effectively in the future.

We smiled, shook hands, and left. Ron now had his marching orders. I don't know if Mother ever knew that Ron had been put on notice. But her account performed much better in subsequent years.

One of the drawbacks to being the peacemaker and best-loved child for John was that he ended up having a tremendous amount of financial responsibility and stress. He willingly shouldered these responsibilities, and was able to manage things amazingly well then, and for the years to come.

We were fortunate in that the three of us agreed about priorities for Mother's care, and we took good care of her money. Actually, we took better care of her funds than we did of our own (self-care can be an issue with many of us). If siblings don't agree, or people undercut one another, then developing a plan can be a real problem.

Reflection: Dealing with Money Matters

No matter what your loved one's financial situation might be, there are things that you will want to do to safeguard their finances, if you can. The sooner you can discuss these issues, the easier it will be to develop and implement a plan. Go ahead, dive in. The water may not be fine, but most of us can navigate it, with help.

There are many more scammers around today than in the early 2000s, when we were dealing with Mother's finances. Scammers can be so wily and sophisticated that the best of them do quite well financially. They can contact older adults by phone, text, email, mail, or, sometimes, in person. Some scammers pretend to be government agencies with names and logos that seem quite official. People may call pretending to be a bank representative, someone from Social Security or Medicare, the IRS, or another official person.

The scams are difficult to address when we find ourselves in the middle of conversations. So, the best defense is a good offense. Talk about the issues with your loved one. Check with the local Senior Center to see if there are workshops on how to avoid scams. Do your own research. Talk about situations that you know about, with friends or other family members, and remember to share those stories.

There are a number of articles about finances and aging that I recommend. A Google search can put you in touch with New York Times articles, Pew research, the University of Pittsburgh Aging Institute as well as regular columns on a number of websites. It seems like financial management skills are some of those affected early in the progression of dementia, and the consequences can be devastating.

As money management becomes more difficult for the elderly with Alzheimer's or dementia, there are a number of things that one can do.

1. *Discuss their goals, priorities, and preferences as soon as possible.*
2. *Build a plan to protect their assets, working with someone who is knowledgeable about finances (financial expert, resources provided through a local Senior Center, faith community, or a family member skilled with finances).*
3. *Develop a list of important documents and their locations (medical insurance, will, health care directives, Power of Attorney, mortgage papers or property deed, bank and brokerage records, etc.). Ensure that list is filed at the house, bank or brokerage safe, and with one or two trusted family members or friends.*
4. *Create a Health Care Limited Power of Attorney (POA) for a trusted family member or friend to serve as the health care resource and shared decision-maker in the event that your loved one cannot make decisions. Involve your loved one as much as possible. The limits ensure that the POA isn't overly broad and defines the roles and responsibilities of the person who will be sharing in and taking over some of the decision-making for your loved one. Whenever possible, the person should be someone you trust, who understands your loved one's preferences, and who will seek to honor those in their healthcare decisions.*
5. *Create a Financial Limited Power of Attorney for a trusted family member or friend to serve as a financial resource for decisions and financial decisions using guidelines similar to those listed above.*
6. *Where possible, protect assets by placing them in joint custody, transfer upon death agreements, and/or trusts. For something this complicated, it is worth seeking the advice of a financial planner who is well-vetted, trusted, and who comes with strong recommendations. Sometimes, financial planners provide free services through Senior Centers, faith communities, or as part of their ongoing work.*

7. *Research care needs, options, and costs and develop plans. Talk with friends or family members who have gone through this before. Find out about agencies that serve older adults in your community and schedule a phone call or meeting with staff to see what resources they have available and know about in the community.*
8. *Check to see what services your loved one's health insurance covers. Research the best possible Medicare plans if they are covered through Medicare. AARP provides excellent information, resources, and referrals about Medicare, as do many local Senior Centers. One challenge in the US is that Medicare does not provide many of the needed in-home services. Many people on limited incomes find they must spend down in order to qualify for Medicaid. That issue is important to discuss with trusted professionals.*
9. *If funds are limited, research options such as reverse mortgages, county and state social service and health care programs, and other benefits to which a parent may be entitled. Local Senior Centers can be excellent resources as you begin your search, as are faith communities, older adult online networks that are run by trusted nonprofits and leaders in the field, and friends that may have shared a similar journey.*

You may find it helpful to consult a professional in a nonprofit such as your local Senior Center that works with the elderly. Talk with financial and tax specialists if you can.

If your loved one has cash assets in the bank and investments, please take special care to protect these assets from scams, or lapses that come with dementia. It is also important to research how to legally and ethically spend down if assets are limited and parents could qualify for Medicaid at some point.

Review your own potential financial liabilities as well. Adult children have more legal issues and potential liabilities now than was the case in the mid to late 1990s and early 2000s, when my mother was dealing with Alzheimer's.

When in doubt, talk with others who have cared for an elderly parent and worked through some of the financial challenges. Make sure that the advice you receive is from people that are well-informed and unencumbered by financial self-interest. You want objective feedback from people in the know.

Chapter 5: Standing Up to Others

Mother was raised in the Deep South, and like most Southern girls, she learned her lessons early. By the time she was grown, she had fully internalized the tenets of being "A Southern Lady," with all of the attendant attitudes, benchmarks, privileges, management skills, and knowledge of accessorizing that are part of that fine art form. She also learned a great deal about how to be tough when situations warranted, standing up for what one believes, and taking charge when needed.

Her mother was a wonderful artist, often disorganized and forgetful. Gram was also a pragmatist, and a fascinating mix of Edwardian Era culture, early feminism, Unity Christianity, and Women's Christian Temperance Union (WCTU) values that go way back to the turn of the century – into 1900, the 1930s and '40s, and beyond! All of these had a significant impact on my mother.

Race Riots in Guam

Mama worked for the Red Cross as a Club Director during the final years of World War II. After a train trip across the country in 1945 to the West Coast, she had an orientation in Honolulu. From there, she went to Guam for a short orientation and training. Then, she was posted on the tiny island of Tinian to run the 'Swabbie Lobby' Recreation Club. These clubs were managed by the Red Cross and scattered throughout the Pacific. They were probably the only place where military personnel had a chance to rest, play, and practice living "the normal life" in the midst of death and destruction that washed over the Pacific and many of them.

Mother's arrival came just a few months after a disastrous race riot in Guam, in late 1944. This riot between African American and White military men resulted in deaths and injuries in Guam, which served as the "hub" for many of the smaller islands, like Tinian.

Both African American and White military came to the Swabbie Lobby Club for food, music, games, skits, reading – and especially for pool. African Americans were often the first to drop by the club because of the way that shifts were scheduled, often around racial lines, as the units were segregated by race. The African Americans were almost always given the worst shifts, those that started very early and ended in the mid-afternoon. Many would head over to the club to play pool after work.

One day, soon after Mother arrived to run the club, some White Army Airmen came in right before dinner. The pool tables were all taken by African Americans who were engrossed in their games. A number of the Airmen were "Good Ole Southern Boys." As such, they felt entitled and unwilling to wait, especially under those circumstances. They came up to Mama saying: "Get those N... out of here."

Instantly, pool playing stopped. The air was electrified, with an explosion just seconds away. Mother had to have been briefed about the earlier race riot in Guam and the dangerous situation that still existed. But with no hesitation, she moved to stand in between the two groups that were fast forming, and said: "I'm from Alabama, and I know as well as anybody how things are done in the South. But we're on an island in the middle of the Pacific Ocean. And we're all in this war together."

Mother was movie-star beautiful at that age, but looked much younger than she was and spoke with a Deep Southern accent. That meant that she needed to ramp up on her authority, because otherwise, the guys could easily walk all over her. She was still naïve about a lot of things, but not all things. Young as she was, she already had that force of personality that characterized her later life.

It was a blend of Southern sweetness and steel. She could claim total control of a volatile situation in a few heartbeats. "I may look young, but I'm older than most of you, and carry a GS rank equivalent of a captain. I run this club. Both groups will stay. Those are the rules."

They were dumbstruck. It was a knock-out.

The Great, Great Dane

During Thanksgiving of 1965, when we were living in San Juan, Mother took my two brothers and me to St. Thomas for the holidays. I'm not sure what preoccupied Dad at the time, perhaps the aftermath of the evacuation of refugees from the Dominican Republic. Whatever it was, he was not in the picture. It was Mother and the three of us.

Mama would spend hours researching each site on our itinerary, so that she would know about the area's history, art, and culture. As I write this, I realized that I have developed the same habit, which has greatly enriched my travels. So often, as we care for elderly loved ones and reflect on the experience, we find that we've adopted some of their characteristics. Depending upon what they are, they can become little treasures or sticking points.

As was her habit when traveling, we started early and spent our days nonstop sightseeing. I loved Charlotte Amalie's sights, the harbor, and the little stores. Already I had learned the fine art of shopping. The scenery was a breathtaking explosion of tropical color. One of the sights tucked away from most tourists was Bluebeard's Castle. It was on private property and very nicely hidden at the end of a residential street. Later, it became a boutique hotel.

As we wound our way up a hill filled with large residential homes, we children began to mutter and complain. We had pretty much had our fill of walking, and this appeared to be a "wild goose chase." However, as the tall and partially ruined tower soon came into view, Mother marched ahead, ready for another of her touring conquests.

Then, out of nowhere, came the largest dog I had ever seen. An enormous Great Dane was leaping over the wall, heading right for us. The size of a small horse (forget pony), the dog was barking ferociously, and would be upon us in just a few bounds. This was one of those times I was so frightened that I literally could not move. I just stared at death on four paws.

Quickly, Mama ran forward, waving her arm and pointing at the dog, saying, "You stop, right now. Go back. Leave these children alone." Once she got the dog's attention, she continued to reprimand it. The dog slowed down and then stopped. About the same time, a woman came out of the house and began calling the dog by some sort of ridiculous name like "Precious" or "Bumpkins."

Hearing his name and her voice, the dog turned around to face her, and with a faint whimper of recognition, bounded back home. I don't remember ever being so proud of Mother, or so grateful that she was there in full spiritual battle armor looking out for us.

Protecting Her Mama

Gram, our grandmother, was in the hospital in her last few days. Born in 1882, Gram was three months shy of 100 years old, and had lived a rich and full life. Even though managed care wasn't yet in its heyday, doctors and hospitals were already glimpsing financial opportunity, and expanding their services to the insured.

This practice developed partly because technology was starting to allow hospitals to provide more options for patients, partly a risk-management measure to avoid lawsuits, and partly to expand billings and increase revenues. Today, after several decades of this policy, we find that the greatest medical expenditures for people are during their last thirty days of life, often due to extensive and unneeded medical heroics.

Whatever the cause, a very young doctor was trying to talk with my exhausted and exasperated mother. He wanted to intubate Grandmother and put her on a respirator. Mother, the daughter of a doctor, had her own ideas. She would not stand by to have her mother's last days or hours stretched out to a near vegetative state. Her father and mother had instilled in her (and in us) a respect for the natural cycle of life without the imposition of extraordinary measures, especially at the end of a very long life. At ninety-nine, Gram had caught pneumonia and was ready to go.

The rather clueless doctor was working hard, trying to chip away at Mother's resolve, using his newfound status as an appointed medical god (with a little "G"). Finally, Mother had had enough, and she lambasted the unwitting guy with unexpected fury.

"Now you listen here, young man," Mother said to him, shaking her finger at him for emphasis and effect. "My father was a doctor, with a great deal more experience than you have now at your tender age. We value life, but we don't believe in these unnecessary tactics to prolong life, especially at her age."

The doctor was aghast and continued to press his point. Mother was unimpressed. "Young man, if this were your grandmother, would you suggest that course of treatment? Knowing she's at the end of her life? A very full life?" She looked down her nose at the young MD.

He was backing down and literally backing off as she kept going at him. She continued to press her point and her finger at his face, so that he literally backed all the way down the hall. She frog-marched him backward for a good while. "I will not stand for extraordinary measures. I won't allow it. My mind is made up, and you will not change it. Now leave us alone."

The doctor left, but not without first giving Mother a referral slip for a psychiatrist. There were many times we three children felt that sort of referral would have been appropriate and helpful. Just not then. Thank goodness Mother had the strength to prevail against the turkey in the white coat.

Game, set, and match to Mother. When she was good, she was very, very good.

Reflection: At the Core

It was important for me to understand and reflect on what was quintessentially "Mama." At her core.

That essence was deeply ingrained in her values, attitudes, and habits. It continued to guide her actions and way of responding to what Alzheimer's was doing to her.

She fought hard and stood her ground. That allowed her to persevere in many ways. It also made things very difficult during her early stages, as she fought so many of our efforts.

We were amazed and deeply respected her grit.

It was also exhausting.

That was Mama.

Chapter 6: A Change to Her Summer Visit

During the spring of 1997, my brothers and I became increasingly concerned about Mother's care. I was going to Winston-Salem about four times a year, and Tom and John were covering the other months. But we were afraid it was no longer sufficient. We were sharing the management of her care (such as it was), with each of us handling certain aspects.

John was handling her banking, brokerage accounts, and taxes. After we updated her will with her, he had Power of Attorney over her financial affairs. He was working on his PhD at the University of Kansas, and went to see Mother about every other month. Tom was in Louisville. Both had heavy teaching schedules, but were somehow able to ensure that one of them was with her for about a week every month, with me filling in during spring, summer, and winter holidays.

Tom and his wife Ann worked on keeping the house itself in shape and helping to retain help, or re-hire people she had told weren't needed.

I worked on revising her will and researching options for her care.

The three of us worked as a team, and actually agreed about most things, which I realized in retrospect was a huge gift. That level of agreement about core values and goals made everything much easier than it might have been otherwise.

I offered to take Mother to Santa Fe for the summer. It seemed like that was only fair, since I had not visited her in Winston-Salem as often as had Tom and John. My brothers did need a break. It appeared that I would be able to handle my clients and care for Mother. In fact, I thought she might enjoy the summer music, the opera, and the arts. She loved the mountains, and we had plenty of those. Last time I checked, the Sangre de Cristos are still there, still awe-inspiring.

We arranged for Mama to have a check-up with her doctor to make sure that she could handle the trip. The doctor indicated that, other than the dementia, she was in good health and would be fine to travel and spend time in the high altitude of the Santa Fe mountains.

In early June, I flew to pick up Mother and bring her back with me to Santa Fe. We had handled the reservations for the return trip for the two of us very carefully, to minimize the time in transit, and to ensure arrival in New Mexico before dark.

When we arrived at the airport, we were informed the flight had been either canceled or delayed. Mother's Alzheimer's had progressed at this point, and she was suffering from moderate memory loss. We knew that travel would be dicey with the best possible scenario, much less a major roadblock.

My sister-in-law and I demanded to talk with a manager and explained Mother's condition. He made the usual excuses, at which point I used all of the strategies I had learned from Mama to "read him the riot act," as she would have said.

Ann and I knew that if we didn't leave then, it would be much more difficult to return to the house, only to try and depart again later. It might not happen at all, or with extreme difficulty. We were looking at a window that was fast narrowing, and we needed to take action. We demanded and received a ticket for the next available flight from another carrier, and so began our journey for Mother's summer vacation with me.

We all learned some very important lessons from that exchange with the airline manager. We realized that normal travel inconveniences for most of us become huge life-changing obstacles when dealing with Mama, who was not frail, with Alzheimer's disease. We had spent days, weeks, and months preparing for the trip, getting Mother ready and packed. A long wait or reschedule for the next day could have jettisoned all of our plans.

We learned that, when necessary, one should demand to speak with a manager and expect reasonable accommodation. We also learned about the importance of having an advocate. By teaming up, Ann and I had greater resolve and capacity than either of us would have had alone.

After we received our new tickets, Ann said to me: "Boy, I would not have wanted to be in his shoes. You were something else." I smiled at Mama, thinking that this was a set of skills I had learned from her starting at an early age. They were very well ingrained, sometimes too much so.

Our trip west required a stopover and change of planes in Denver. In fact, it's difficult to fly from the East Coast to New Mexico without changing planes. There were a few options, but most were nonstop from Albuquerque to Atlanta, Baltimore, or Orlando. There were no nonstop flights from Winston-Salem to Albuquerque or Santa Fe. So, we carefully planned for a little extra time in Denver. It would be a long trip for anyone, much less Mama with Alzheimer's.

The flight went well, and we had a nice dinner in Denver. I had arranged for a wheelchair, which Mother found insulting. However, the walk would have been impossible for her, and she would have been confused by the people-movers that zipped along in the center of the terminals.

So, I told Mama that they were offering wheelchairs to many passengers at that point, as part of a training program for new staff, and that it would be very helpful to the airline if she were willing to help out. In that case, she agreed, and we were off to make our connection.

Over time, I continued to develop a gift for making things up, or lying on the spot, when needed.

The woman who was pushing the wheelchair was from Mexico, and she was absolutely wonderful with Mother. No matter what Mother said, she responded in a compassionate and respectful way. Unlike so many, she was not embarrassed or challenged by Mother's dementia and her wild chatter. I thanked her and talked with her from time to time in Spanish about her move to the US and her dreams. I let her know how much I appreciated the way she dealt with Mother. She had made the transition much easier, and I gave her a large tip in gratitude.

The airline policy of boarding people with special needs first was and is a tremendous help. We got Mother situated and thought we would be off. However, there was a delay. For some reason, we waited on the tarmac for long enough for Mother to become distressed and agitated. By this time, it was late afternoon. Mother had not had her nap. She was tired, increasingly agitated, and becoming a bit difficult. We all can get a bit difficult when exhaustion and frustration hit at the end of a long day. She was wondering why we couldn't get going.

"Anne Hays, why aren't we moving?" she asked repeatedly. The flight attendant was wonderful, asking her if she wanted something cold to drink, which she did. But Mama continued her queries, becoming a bit more upset. When I talked about the plane, she didn't seem to understand. So, I finally hit on a good answer. "Mama, we're waiting for the train to leave the station. The train will be leaving any minute now." She sat back, pleased to finally understand what was happening.

A man sitting nearby gave me a number of nasty stares. He seemed irritated by Mother's constant worried banter and gave me a dirty look soon after I talked about the train. I finally glared at him in response and thought that expression might convey my irritation at him for his haughtiness. Perhaps he got my message of: "Look, it worked. She has Alzheimer's. Give it a rest. Perhaps you'll get the opportunity for hands-on learning yourself someday." And so forth.

Finally, we arrived in Albuquerque, both exhausted. As we began to de-plane, the flight attendant mentioned to us that a wheelchair was waiting for Mother. To which Mother replied, "Oh yes, she had one of those for me before. But I'm not nearly as old and frail as she thinks."

Then she winked and smiled at the flight attendant as she walked off with a flourish. The flight attendant and I had a moment where our eyes connected, and she seemed to say "Good luck." It helped.

We had a nice ride up to Santa Fe, and Mother loved seeing the mountains in the early evening light. She was treated to her first of two beautiful sunsets over the Sangre de Cristo Mountains that encircle Santa Fe. Once we arrived at my house, we had dinner. She played with the cat and we talked about Santa Fe. She played my piano a little, and then we both turned in. It had been an exhausting day.

The days to come were to be even more stressful.

The next morning, I awoke refreshed and ready to go. Mother was still sleeping, so I tried to keep quiet. But, after a few hours of intermittent checking on her, I finally brought her some breakfast.

She woke extremely dizzy and was not able to keep anything down. She went back to sleep. I called my friend Beth, who was a nurse. She recommended I keep an eye on things, try to get her to eat, and to call her back if Mother didn't improve. After repeated attempts, trying a number of things, I began to worry that she might not be getting enough oxygen or liquids, and that she could become increasingly dehydrated.

After some effort, I was able to get Mother dressed, but she went back to bed again, saying, "I'll feel better soon. I've just got such a woozy head. Do you have any smelling salts?" Fortunately, I found some, and they helped a little, but not much. She had not eaten since the previous evening, and had very little to drink. She lay back down again.

I called Beth again. She said that she and her husband would come over and help me get Mother to the hospital emergency room. Beth and Chris were wonderful. She and her husband came over right away. We tried to get Mama to walk between us, but she was stumbling. Beth's husband, Chris, said to me, "She's so small, I can carry her." And, to Mother, he asked, "Do you mind if I carry you to the car?"

Waving one hand as if she had a lace handkerchief, she smiled as he was picking her up. Never one to miss an entrance or exit, she said "Oh, my. You're so strong. You're such a nice young man." Off they went, with Beth and me in tow.

At the hospital, we discovered that her oxygenation levels had dropped to the high 80 percent level, so she was given oxygen there and a prescription for an oxygen tank. Relieved, we packed her up and took her back to my house. Soon, we were equipped with a portable oxygen tank, and I began to think we had solved the problem.

Not so.

Later, when I went in to check on Mother, she had taken off the oxygen tube. I started to fix it for her and she complained, "Oh, Anne Hays, I can't stand this. It scratches my nose. It's awful." As I explained how important it was for her to use to breathe, she seemed to understand and agreed to wear it. She lay back down. After a few more minutes, I checked on her again. She was napping comfortably, without the oxygen. This went on for a few hours. I would fix it, and she would take it off.

I finally realized that, with her dementia, she would probably not be able to remember to keep the oxygen tube attached. Consequently, her blood oxygenation would drop, and she would continue to have altitude sickness.

I called both brothers and explained what was happening. We all agreed that Mama would probably not do well in Santa Fe after all. We planned for me to return her back home. We were able to book a flight the next day. Fortunately, I was able to keep her hydrated, oxygenated, and fed enough that she was able to avoid becoming dizzy and ill again. So, as luck would have it, we were able to travel the next day.

I called the airline and spent quite a bit of time setting things up so that someone would meet the car with a wheelchair while I took the car to short-term parking and came back around. That was not to be, and the departure turned into a circus.

Once we dropped below the 7,200-foot elevation of Santa Fe, Mama started to feel a bit better, which was a good thing since she continued to remove her oxygen tube. But even though she was feeling better, she was still weak and would not be able to walk more than a few steps. I thought that the pre-arranged wheelchair would solve that problem. I arrived, but the wheelchair was not there. Thus started a very challenging trip to return Mother back home. Once at the airport, she quickly became tired, and the trip was long, difficult, and confusing for her. It was for me, too.

I was both relieved and upset to be returning Mama back home. We had done everything we could to check out the trip beforehand, including a conversation with her doctor. But I still felt somewhat guilty for not being able to care for her as well as my brothers had done, and felt somehow responsible for the "failed summer trip."

Later, I was to realize that many medical professionals are quite limited in their understanding of how high altitude affects the elderly, especially those that have lived for many years at sea level. It may be that medical professionals are challenged when it comes to discussing a frail elderly parent's condition and limitations within different environments. Things are better than they were in the mid to late 1990s, but the health care system needs a great deal of improvement if we are to effectively address the growing challenges facing this next group of older adults now retiring. Baby boomers like me.

That experience, and many others like it, taught me to always do my own research in addition to checking with medical professionals, financial and legal advisers, and others. It also taught me to have a support system in place that I could depend upon when the inevitable surprises would come my way. In this case, my brothers were expecting to have a summer off and I was not anticipating Mother's serious altitude sickness. We were able to manage the changes because we had support networks in place and were willing to be flexible. I spent additional time with Mama in Louisville, and my brothers and sister-in-law pitched in.

Oftentimes, a friend who has recently cared for an elderly parent can be a godsend. My friend Nancy's mother had died a few years before, and she was in a position where she could talk about the challenges and the good times with a bit of objectivity. Her stories buoyed me and gave me perspective. I talked with a number of other friends and often with my two brothers. This helped us to think about different options, consider new strategies, and get support for the stressful work of caring for an elderly parent.

From this and so many other experiences with Mama, I learned to plan as well as possible, develop support, and be ready for the unexpected. Expect it!

For us, it was a wild ride.

Reflection: Dealing with Unexpected Challenges

It can be so frustrating to spend hours developing a plan for some area of an elderly loved one's care, to then see things go up in smoke! Whether it's a parent, spouse, sibling, or other loved one, it's challenging. I was frustrated and angry. Later, I realized that we all did the best we could with the information we had.

The doctor indicated that even with Mother's history of lung problems, she would be fine in Santa Fe. The problem was, the doctor didn't really know what he was talking about. He didn't understand the impact of high-altitude living on elderly people. Many elderly people find that they cannot handle the thin air at Santa Fe's altitude of between 7200 and 7800 feet above sea level.

What can you do?

Plan as best you can. Research any area related to travel with or moving a frail elderly parent. Talk with others who have encountered similar situations.

Then develop a backup plan. One thing you can count on is that some of your plans won't work – for all kinds of reasons. It's part of what makes caring for an elderly parent frustrating and sometimes scary. We really are not in control much of the time.

Try to limit the number of variables you must deal with. Give yourself plenty of time and add extra time on top of that just to give yourself a bit more "wiggle room." Build in some support for yourself so that you can take care of yourself while you're also taking care of your loved one.

If you get hit with the hard edge of the unexpected and realize you're caught in a bind, ask for help.

Chapter 7: Hiring, Firing, and Blowing Smoke

As we began to spend more time with Mama, we realized that she needed additional help at home to manage day-to-day chores. For some time, we had continued to keep the yard man that Dad had hired years ago. Since she knew him and was comfortable with him, Mama was fine having Bill come to work in the yard. She had help in the house for many years, but for some reason, there had been nobody to help out for a number of years and Mama was trying to manage the house, which was too hard for her. It was painful to see all that she couldn't manage, and a dirtier house. We pitched in so that the house was clean, groceries stocked up, and repairs made whenever we visited, but it wasn't enough.

We wanted to jump in to make things all better.

Our solution was to "help" Mama by hiring a housekeeper. The first few times we hired someone; she acted as if she were in full agreement. Someone would be hired to come in to clean and make sure that Mama was all right. But always, within a week or so after we'd left, the person we hired would be gone. Nothing we tried seemed to help.

For someone with diminished mental capacity, Mama was extremely clever when she wanted or needed to be. Mother would say something like: "Oh, I'm not sure what happened. I think she got another job," or "I'm all by myself. It's just me, and I don't have to have someone to clean up after me. It's a nuisance." She would often complain that it was too expensive and that she just didn't have that kind of money anyway. She may have been afraid and we didn't realize it and didn't know how to handle it.

About money. As adults who came of age during the Great Depression, our parents were so tight with their money that it sometimes screamed in protest. The feeling of not having enough permeated their psyches, and they passed along some of that to the three of us.

The truth was that the two of them had lived frugally all of their lives, scrimping, saving, and investing wisely. When we were growing up, we hardly ever went out to eat, and when we did, it was usually the occasional trip to Morrison's Cafeteria after church. Mother sewed her clothes and mine to save money. She loved it. I hated it. I wanted the clothes with the labels. The Villagers and the sweaters with the ribbons down the front of them. The Weejuns.

They liked the "Blue Light Specials" at Kmart. They splurged little, but when they did, it was on a lovely house in a neighborhood full of large lawns and big trees. They saved like crazy for our college funds, music lessons and concerts, books, and travel. Over the years, they had managed very well in spite of their fears and control issues.

Now, in her old age, Mother had a nice nest egg. Not enough to live a wanton high life. But more than enough to cover her needs.

However, the financial fears and frugality were so deeply ingrained that she knew no other reality. In fact, we realized later that as her grasp of reality slipped in her final years, she lived in fear of impoverishment. Getting her to accept help was an uphill battle at best.

My brother John, the one who visited most often, was tasked with making sure she was able to manage in the house. He worked to keep scheduling supports like the housekeeper/caregiver. Whenever he met with the inevitable next prospective housekeeper, he made sure to explain to the caregiver that he was the one hiring, and to Mama the importance of having this help around the house.

"That will take care of things," we thought. These extra times with conversations with both Mama and the housekeeper/caregiver would reduce the endless cycle of churning through different people.

We thought, at this juncture, that she understood that she could afford and deserved this expenditure. It appeared she had deferred to his wishes. When talking about it later, he remembered that she smiled and told him how much she appreciated our concern. "You are so good to me, but you worry too much. Your old Mother has been taking care of herself for a lot longer than you have, you know."

Left-handed compliments were her specialty. She also had mastered the art form of appearing to defer to others and then doing what she wanted anyway. But she hardly ever really deferred. She just pretended to. Mama liked being in control, especially as control over her own world was slipping. She was very crafty and knew how to get her way, as do many Southern women. After all, that culture has relegated them to the margins when it comes to direct action, and many excel at the use of indirect power.

Mama explained: "The neighbors are like family. They take me grocery shopping and sometimes to the mall. Louise picks me up for church. I still drive some, you know. Not on the big roads, but to get music and so forth." Her comment "and so forth" would become one of the many expressions she would use more often over time to mask her diminishing vocabulary.

A very deep bond had formed between Mother and the couple next door some years ago when their teenager was a baby. Mary had gone back to work and had someone full-time looking after the baby. The childcare worker was not to take him out anywhere in her car, but she did. Mother noticed. She told Mary about the lapse so that Mary could take action right away. They were like family after that.

Not only were the neighbors incredibly helpful to Mother during the last few years, they provided us with updates on her condition and how they saw her coping. They also provided Mother with a great smokescreen she used often with us when she felt we were interfering too much (which, unfortunately, was often). She'd let us know that they were always around, grocery shopping and helping out with little things that were now too difficult for her to handle.

When we could, we'd hire people for a short while, and then Mama would fire them. That became ritualized into a dance that occupied a fair amount of all of our time. It did until we realized that we just needed to prioritize things, and let the low-priority issues alone. We had to learn to let certain things slide. Following repeated failures, we stopped putting so much effort into the task of finding her a housekeeper.

We were to learn that caring for an elderly parent with Alzheimer's required constant prioritizing, along with a willingness to let go of those things that can be postponed, which are not critical. Those skills became lifelines for us later on.

We were also worried about Mama's driving, especially after she told us that she only used the car for short trips, like to the music store, always avoiding "the big roads." The big roads, we discovered, referred to the two interstates that bisected Winston-Salem. She had never liked driving on the interstate, but had not called it "the big road" until after we noticed her problems with her memory.

We were to learn many times over the years that, despite the gradual diminution of her mental capacity, her ability to take control to do things her way was not diminished to the same extent. Nor was her musical memory. She may have become more committed to getting her way as one method of controlling her world, which was fast becoming smaller, less predictable, and much more confusing. She was sliding into Alzheimer's, and, at some level, she may have realized that and was fighting it with everything she had.

Her driver's license was coming up for renewal. Naively, we thought that, with her memory problems, she might not even notice the license expiration date. We figured she would simply let her license lapse.

We were wrong. She definitely noticed, and she was determined to keep her license. Again, this represented an important part of being an independent adult. She told us not to worry, that she would handle things. And handle them she did.

Mother contacted Louise, her friend who always took her to church. She asked Louise to take her to get her license renewed. There were so many times when Mother was confused about her music schedule, or billing, or her bank balance. But she knew she needed to renew her license, and it was a priority for her.

Louise and my brother John were quite close, so she called him to tell him about the license renewal. Interestingly, Mother had not mentioned this to any of us. As Louise and John talked, they both figured that Mother would fail the test, and that would be the end of that. So, nobody was really worried about Mother's driving at that point.

A few days later, Louise called John in hysterics. "You would not believe what your mother did this morning," she said.

John was afraid that perhaps there had been a scene, or Mother had become upset at not having her license renewed. But that wasn't it at all. Louise explained that Mother had been dressed and ready to go when she arrived to pick her up. And Mother arrived at the Motor Vehicle Department battle ready.

With the skill of any hardened general, Mother had planned her attack and executed her strategies brilliantly. She chatted up the man who was giving her the paper and pencil test, flirting and telling him how smart he was, and asking for definitions to some of the questions.

Even with early Alzheimer's, she had still managed to outfox the clerk and get him to give her answers to many of the questions without his having any idea he was doing that.

"I couldn't believe it," said Louise. "Here she was, just talking away, and getting one answer after another. When I picked her up, I could tell she was ready for that test. She was really something else. And she knew exactly what she was doing! In fact, she said to me as we left, 'Now wasn't that just the nicest young man.'"

John and Louise had a good laugh, and then he called me and our brother Tom to give us the bad news: Mama still had a valid driver's license. In our next phone conversations with her, she let each of us know that, "yes, of course I got my license renewed."

She crowed a bit and was quite pleased with herself, if the truth be told. She had a right to be proud. She had emerged victorious this time in one of her many little battles with her brain.

We realized we needed to do something to keep our eyes on her driving, and try to get her to either not drive or to limit her activities. But she would change the subject often when we discussed driving. We began watching the odometer on her car. It didn't move. For months, it didn't move.

We'd ask her about driving, couching our questions in not so cleverly disguised queries about how well the car was performing, and whether it needed any maintenance work. She would almost always respond by saying something like: "It's just fine. I don't drive that much. But it's a good solid car."

In fact, for most of that year, the odometer showed no movement. So, after a while, my brother John decided to remove one of the spark plugs to keep her from driving. We were all afraid that driving once in a great while would be much more dangerous than not driving at all. Having the car not start could serve as an important barrier to driving without impinging upon her sense of independence and self-agency. We felt like cheats, but it seemed like the right thing to do.

Mama never talked with us about not being able to start the car. And we never mentioned driving to her again.

We realized later that she felt so much more comfortable and in control by having a current driver's license and a car in the garage. Never mind that she never used the car anymore. It was a symbol. And at some level she was sharp enough to realize that she needed the symbols (the license and the car). She also must have realized at some level that driving was becoming more difficult and dangerous for her.

In spite of her advancing Alzheimer's, she was smart, savvy, and sassy. This probably helped her during the early stages of that difficult journey that none of us can fully understand what it's like to be caught living in.

But what we did not see at that point was her gradual withdrawal from others. She went to church less often. She had been sick, so we thought the change was due to her health. However, as time went on, she went to church less and less.

For years, she had been a leader in the church, active with Presbyterian Women and other groups. But her connections waned and she began to make excuses. "Well, last Sunday, I was just tired," or "You know, it's not the same," or even "Perhaps I'll go next week." Even when Louise would offer to come and pick her up and sit with her, Mother made one excuse after another.

She became increasingly unwilling to engage in social activity, especially on a large scale like a church service. Louise began coming over a bit more often to visit with Mother and talk about church activities, which she enjoyed a great deal.

Mama had been the President of the local chapter of the Music Teachers Association, but by this time she had few contacts with that network. She had a very few students, three I think, who she taught most weeks until the late 1990s. She practiced and played for her own enjoyment. And she talked about music with her sister, Tula, who taught piano as well as violin.

Music had been, and continued to be, a large part of Mama's life. She played well and practiced her favorite pieces faithfully. There was little change evidenced in that sphere of her life. She continued to look for new music for her students. Even with the final three students, she worked to supplement *John Thompson's Book Three* with fun pieces like *Golliwog's Cake Walk* and *The Elephant.*

Even after she fully retired from teaching, she still played the piano every day. She played until about two weeks before she died of severe Alzheimer's. We marveled at the power of musical memory in her life.

A parent with Alzheimer's disease provides grown children with many surprises. The trajectory of the disease is like a sailboat tacking across a large body of water in variable weather conditions. There is a great deal of change in one's condition and in one's ability to navigate.

Sometimes, our loved one surprises us with their skill, abilities, and acuity, as Mother did with the trip to the Motor Vehicle Bureau to get her license. We would have never imagined that she could have passed the test. She wouldn't have passed without the unwitting help of "that nice young man." We found it to be hysterically funny, and quintessentially Mother. And she was extremely proud of herself.

Discovering those "islands of competence," and helping point our loved one to those can be an important way of grounding them and us. Alzheimer's advances, it seems, in fits and starts. In the early stages, I believe that many people retain some gifts or skills, and helping them ground in those may be one of the most life-giving of things we do together with them.

Then there are always those times when we discover that things are not going well. We discover new areas of loss, and new challenges.

We saw Mother becoming increasingly confused with handling finances, her billing, and her taxes. We discovered that she was alone more often and becoming isolated. With respect to some of those losses, we thought there were things we could do, and we tried and succeeded at some of them. With others, there was not much we felt we could do, except to visit more often and work to try to build a support network around her.

When one solution failed, like hiring housekeepers, we had learned to let go of our plans and regroup, or try other ideas. Helping Mother deal with life as she began to lose ground required all of the creativity we had.

This was as true for Mother as it was for the three of us. There were things that made us laugh and difficulties that we found sad and disheartening. It was difficult to see someone who had a razor-sharp mind become increasingly befuddled and unable to cope.

That was probably why Mother was so proud of herself in getting her driver's license renewed. It was a triumph.

Dealing with the disease was also exhausting. My brothers and I talked with one another often, increased our visits to her, and helped her manage a more difficult lifeload and workload. We noticed the toll that the additional activity brought, but what we didn't see until later was the stress created by having a loved one with Alzheimer's. She struggled, and we all struggled with her.

We were also beginning to talk about the future, and the options that might exist for her care when she became increasingly unable to cope. But we knew that was still in the future.

The not-too-distant future.

Reflection: Dealing with Resistance

Dealing with a loved one's resistance can be difficult and emotionally draining. A lot often goes into the standoffs.

As middle-aged adults who had been watching Mama lose her financial acumen, ability to follow conversations, and her judgment, we often saw ourselves as the ones bringing answers and light. When she fought us, we often tried to convince her.

When that happened, both sides hardened. It took us a while to realize that tactic was not the best one to use.

Nobody likes to be characterized as "that problem person," or somebody who is not able to manage. When we have been smart all of our lives and depended on our mental skills, we can fight like a wildcat to try to keep control.

Mama was a wildcat.

The experience with her driver's license also taught us a thing or two. We realized that she was not unable to function with all tasks all the time. She still had that spark and that desire to persevere.

Gradually, we began to realize that, with Mama, kid gloves, dissembling, and storytelling worked much better than trying to argue the facts. She had won the round with the driver's license, which must have given her some hope, as well as a sense of accomplishment; short-lived though it was.

We learned to pick our battles carefully. The more you understand about your loved one's ways of decision-making, and what they want and need, the easier it will be to work together to address important issues. There's no one right answer. Find what works to keep your loved one safe and supported, and you sane.

Chapter 8: Considering Options for Her Care

After many months of visiting Mother, taking care of her business affairs, and trying to ensure her comfort and safety, we realized that we were slipping the wrong way down an increasingly sharp incline. We were not maintaining. We were losing ground.

Things were getting tougher and more complicated. We were not going to be able to keep helping her from a distance, each of us visiting her once a month or so.

We faced numerous problems.

We had discovered some time before that soon after we would put supports in place, like a housekeeper, she would let them know gently but firmly that she didn't really need them. She just didn't want the help we arranged. If Mother had been willing or able to allow people to come in to help, we would have been able to manage better from a distance. But, as it was, we were all afraid that at any moment, we would get a call from Mary or Louise saying that Mama had fallen, or gotten lost, or had some other problem that came from living alone.

Mother was increasingly isolated and seldom left the house. She was losing touch with people who had been friends for decades. Thank goodness she had Mary and Baird next door, Louise from the church, Tula and her three children.

She became increasingly afraid that she was near penniless. She didn't want to spend any money. We would reassure her that she had sufficient assets, which just made her laugh at us. John continued to manage her finances, taking on increasingly greater responsibilities, and working carefully to try to handle things as Mother would have herself years before, when her mental faculties were more intact.

We could see that Mama was coming to depend much too much on her dear friends and neighbors, Mary and Baird. We, and they, found we were all concerned about that, and John talked frequently and honestly with them about mutual concerns and options.

Like so many middle-aged children who find themselves as caregivers for an elderly parent, we discovered that we had "backed into" the caregiving roles. We had not expected to be traipsing to North Carolina on a regular basis to provide caregiving to Mother. But that's what happened. My sense is that's usually the way most people find themselves caregiving as elderly parents, siblings, or spouses become increasingly frail.

We found that there just weren't enough hours in the day, or enough days in the month to do what we knew had to be done. Thankfully, Mother had a nice-sized nest egg, so we were able to pay for a few services, when she would allow that to happen.

At that juncture, it became clear that before very long, the task of caring for Mother would become impossibly large for us. John and I lived in the West, a good day's trip by plane; and Louisville was a long day's drive for Tom and Ann.

We were each afraid in our own way that something bad could happen to Mama. It didn't matter that she refused a lot of the help that had been offered. We felt individually and collectively responsible for her. Increasingly responsible as her skills diminished.

At this point, we were starting to face a sort of anticipatory guilt for something that might go wrong. It was, quite frankly, an awful feeling.

As the eldest, I have often found myself raising issues with my two brothers when we needed to discuss family matters. And this was no different. I talked with each brother separately and together. When I brought up my concerns about Mother's care, they agreed that she was fast becoming frail and forgetful, and we could all see a time soon when she would not be able to remain in her house alone.

Over the months, I began researching nursing homes and discussed my findings with my brothers. It seemed like the best choice to me at the time, but neither of them was ready to move forward with the decision. They did not want to place her in a facility.

In retrospect, I'm glad that my initial suggestions met with resistance. They were right. We found that out later on when Mother was in a rehabilitation facility for about a month, she drove the staff to distraction with her repetitious questions and demands. In fact, when she told the staff she was ready to leave, they agreed with her that everybody would celebrate that, when it happened!

It's not easy trying to figure out how to care for a frail elderly parent. For one thing, they have their own priorities. Most need to remain as independent as possible. I imagine I will be resistant to efforts for caregiving and making decisions for me when I reach that age.

Mother, with her own unique personality and need for control, was especially resistant to our efforts to help. She actively resisted our best-intended suggestions much of the time.

In some cases, it felt like we had fast backtracked and reverted to how we felt as children. It felt awful! We were hiding some of the things we were doing that we knew Mama didn't like, and telling tales in order to stay out of what we expected would be trouble. We glossed over things in order to avoid her outbursts. That reverting was extremely difficult, as we had our own adverse childhood experiences (ACEs) we'd addressed over the years.

We also found that, even when we were thrown back to those times of feeling like children misbehaving, our roles had very much reversed. We were in that uncomfortable position of parenting our parent. We wanted to do the right thing. We often felt clumsy, incredibly stressed, and ill-prepared to parent her.

Like others going through similar situations, we stumbled along our way to solutions. It was messy. We made a lot of mistakes. We had a lot of successes.

Gradually, as we talked about the challenges, we began to see what would not work more quickly than what would work. And we kept muddling along.

After some time, we realized that we could think of a nursing home as an option, but not the only option. We shared stories and compared notes. Over a period of six to nine months, we handled things by increasing our number of visits, developing a list of things that needed our attention, and dividing up tasks.

Finally, at Christmas that year, we sat down late one evening after Mother went to bed to talk about what in the world we should and could do.

We knew that, although there were a number of options, there were really only a few practical alternatives to consider.

- We could try to put her in a nursing home, but the good ones had long waiting lists, and the costs were high. We knew she would blow her stack at the mere thought of being "put away," and that was not pleasant to contemplate.

- We could leave her in Winston-Salem, but we knew that she would probably have some type of accident or incident – and sooner rather than later.

- We realized that we could have a competency hearing and have one of us declared as her guardian. But she was still sharp enough some of the time to realize what was happening, and we knew that would break her heart.

Quite frankly, the options all looked rather grim. It was hard to think about what to do next at that point. We were tired and extremely stressed.

It was turning out to be a hard Christmas that year.

Reflection: Things That Were Useful for Us

When caring for an elderly parent, most of us face times during the journey when we feel absolutely overwhelmed, stressed, out of control, and helpless. Whatever the challenge, at the time, it usually feels intractable. It's an OMG emergency, huge problem that can't be solved. That's how the overwhelm may feel.

More times than we'd like, it requires more of us than we can give. It is a devastating place to find oneself. Most of us find ourselves in that place at least once during the time we care for our elderly parents. Many of us encounter this multiple times.

So, what can you do? I'll outline some things that we discovered helped, and point out a number of resources that can be of assistance to you no matter what your particular situation.

Here's what we found was useful for us.

1. *Have a Plan. A plan helps, and it can be simple. When we're up against a wall, being able to refer back to a plan is important. A plan serves as an anchor.*

2. *Find and Use Resources. Go to the Alzheimer's Association website, as well as others, such as the National Council on Aging, National Caregiving Association, and the websites for your local Senior Center and other community agencies. Talk with someone at your local Senior Center. You may find new resources you didn't know existed, services that can be scheduled, local respite care programs, faith community support, and volunteers who might be able to help out.*

3. *Prioritize and Clear the Decks.* When times are especially tough, do only what you must. Prioritize your "To Do" list and remove anything that isn't essential. It can be dealt with later.

4. *Create Your Support Team.* Get additional help from family members, friends, and people you've met who have gone through this. Find an Alzheimer's support group. What's too heavy for any one of us can be made lighter when shared. Check with your local or state Alzheimer's Association or Senior Center.

5. *Get Help for the Practical Stuff.* Help with regular caregiving, household tasks, and transportation is often essential. It's not only the mental and emotional stress, but the sheer workload that can be overwhelming. Sit down with your family and friends who are part of your Support Team. Identify the tasks that need to be handled, how they're being handled now, and what needs to be done in the near future. Talk with others who have gone through this caregiving experience for their ideas and suggestions.

6. *Remember, it's Tough for Everyone.* You, your loved one with dementia, family members, and friends. You're all in the soup together. It won't last forever. Crises will come. Crises will go. You will live through it, perhaps with some scars, often with deep appreciation of the sacred space shared.

7. *Take Time for Yourself.* Even if you need to wrestle that time for yourself, do it. Time to take care of yourself is critical. Even if you feel like you don't have five minutes to spare, give yourself four minutes of peace. Meditate for a few minutes if you can. Take deep breaths. Try to give yourself some small gifts of healthy things – time with a friend or family member who lifts your spirits, a favorite book, a walk outdoors, a date night with your spouse or partner. Whatever feeds your soul.

8. *Give Yourself A Little Boost Every Day. Know that your caring for a loved one with dementia is amazing, and you are wonderful. Give yourself some small gift of appreciation every day. Thank yourself in some small way. Give yourself power for the journey.*

Chapter 9: Striking Out and Striking a Bargain

As we moved into the next year, we found that Mama continued to be stubborn about any questions we posed about her health, house, or her independence. That, of course, covered a lot of ground.

Mama had become stubborn about a number of things. Actually, a lot of things. She was never known for her flexibility, and as she struggled with her memory and her fading independence, she became absolutely mulish. When we mentioned we were concerned about her living alone, she would stop the conversation by telling us to change the subject. Sometimes, she would just walk out of the room in a huff.

Mother could still make a dramatic exit when needed.

Feeling in a bit of a quandary, we decided we'd call Mother's sister Tula and talk with her about the situation. We hoped that Tula would have her usual calming effect on Mama. We also hoped somewhat naively that Tula might be able to convince Mama that we were very concerned and were actually trying to help (not punish) her.

So, one evening, we called Tula. It started out as a nice conversation, catching up with one another and trading stories. Southern families love stories, and Gram's branch of the tree was full of storytellers, including Mama, Tula, and many of their children.

After a while, the conversation turned to our concern about Mama, and things went downhill faster than a world-class skier. One minute we were chatting, and the next minute, Mama laid into us, giving us no quarter.

"So, you think your old Mother is crazy?"
"No, Mama," and "No, Lorene," we all said in unison.
"I'll have you know I've lived a lot longer than you children and I know a thing or two. So, you just hush up."

"Now, Lorene. They love you. They're just trying to be helpful," said Tula.

"Tula, you don't know what I have to deal with. They're trying to put me away. I won't have it."

At this point, the conversation had become a shooting match with Mother lined up against the four of us. Though she was outnumbered, she was still in clear command. She was intimidating in spite of her cognitive impairment. Tula assured her that she loved her, and that she knew we meant well.

We all apologized and got off of the phone as soon as possible.

Poor Tula was a wreck. I found out in a quiet call made soon afterward to check on her and to apologize for putting her in the middle of things. We worked hard not to do that again and asked for her help in a big way only one more time later on.

Mother, on the other hand, was on a tear. She stormed around the house in a full tirade. She accused us of calling her crazy, of not minding her, and many other things. Basically, we all sat in the kitchen with our heads down, trying not to agitate her further, and waiting for the storm clouds to subside. They finally passed, but only after a time.

Just as she did when we were children growing up, Mother informed us that although she was very upset with our behavior, she still loved us in spite of the terrible treatment we'd dished out. We said good night. Everyone kissed and made up, and Mama went upstairs to bed.

We, on the other hand, remained down in the kitchen, whispering about the situation and wondering what in the world we would do. We had discussed the options before. Many times.

Not one of the options was good. But this time, we knew that we had finally come to the point where we had to do something. She wasn't safe alone anymore. But she didn't want to do anything we suggested, either.

We were really stuck.

It felt absolutely awful. This time was probably one of the low points for the three of us. We felt at a terrible impasse. We were exhausted, angry, and upset.

We had done our homework and were ready to take some actions that would protect our mother if we absolutely had to do that. But we simply could not think about having us court-ordered to be her guardians. It's hard to feel that helpless.

In addition to feeling helpless, we were all growing increasingly angry at Mama and at the situation. Her resistance was due only partially to her Alzheimer's, and to the normal desire not to lose independence. She had a long history of bad behavior. She could be a drama queen and a willful, intransigent harridan when she felt threatened.

We were stuck in a very difficult stalemate.

We also felt very much afraid as we confronted the situation. Afraid for her. Afraid for ourselves. All three of us are teachers and researchers, so we place a great deal of stock in studying an issue and talking about it. We do love to talk. So, we did.

I went upstairs to check on Mama, to make sure she was in bed. My brothers remained in the kitchen talking in "sotto voce." For the first time I could remember, we were beginning to lose heart. We were afraid that we might have to take legal action to have Mama declared incompetent if we could not find a way to move her to a safer place, closer to one of us or to bring in some serious support for her at home in Winston.

We were still reeling from her tirade prior to the kissee-kissee forgiveness and making up. That combination of tirade followed by making up permeated our lives. From the time we were little to long after we were grown, it was a regular part of our existence.

Mama had let us know in no uncertain terms that she would not consider moving. She was still angry following the lengthy phone call with Tula. She didn't remember a lot of what happened recently, but she could often remember what was most inconvenient for us.

This conversation, unfortunately, she remembered very well.

"I don't know what we're going to do," I said to my brothers. "This is terrible."

"It does not look good," they replied.

We talked for a long time about our options. We were concerned about trying to get conservatorship in North Carolina, when none of us lived in the state. We feared it could be a lengthy and expensive process. We were concerned that she might find a way to rise to the occasion once again and, though she was much less able now to "pass for normal," she could still surprise us. We realized that, if we prevailed, it would break her heart and ours. And it would probably break her spirit.

Even though she had considerable memory loss, she did remember certain things, and she would probably understand part of what was happening to her. We were concerned that it could throw her into a rage, and further off an emotional cliff. We shuddered at the thought of what legal action would do to her and to us. We feared that we didn't have the strength to face something that would undoubtedly be ugly at best.

Like so many adult children caring for a frail, elderly parent, there were many times when we felt overwhelmed by the enormity of the tasks. This was definitely one of those times. There did not seem to be any good options. Only varying levels of difficulty and challenge. So, we decided we'd think about it and continue talking.

Something happened as we talked that can only be called grace.

As we continued our discussion, an idea began to hatch. One of us, probably Tom, came up with a plan that struck all of us as a wonderful, creative, and rather daring solution. This was breakthrough thinking that represented the only decent alternative we could find.

Tom proposed that we talk with Mother about how much he and his wife Ann wanted her to visit because they hadn't seen as much of her as they would like. He suggested we all talk with her about how they needed her to visit and needed her help. We could use this story as a ruse to get her to Louisville, and in a safer, more supervised situation.

We spent some time talking through the strategy. Over the next few days, it continued to take shape. It morphed from an initial idea of a long winter visit to a potential move for Mother. We decided we would look to see if we could find some property very close to Tom and Ann's we could purchase for Mother.

Ann was a real estate broker, and a great help to us in looking at options. Since we had Mother's Financial Power of Attorney, we knew we could purchase a house near Tom and Ann's, if that became our best option.

All of that felt big and scary!

We decided we would take things one step at a time, and grow into whatever would work best. We started with a commitment to plant the seed and talk with Mother about visiting Tom and Ann.

There were a number of times at the beginning that we felt a bit guilty about this level of subterfuge. After all, we were planning to move her from her home in Winston-Salem, where she had lived for over twenty-five years, to the new place in Louisville. However, the neighbors who had been like children to Mother had been talking with us about Mother's recent declines. They were becoming very uncomfortable with being Mama's "go to" help in times of need. They were doing more for Mama than was appropriate, and had needed to rescue her from time to time. It was too much, even for very close friends who were almost like her children.

As Mama's health and memory continued to slip, it caused them, and us, great concern. Her neighbors, Mary and Baird, were both medical professionals and were very worried about her continuing to live in the house alone. She was increasingly at risk, especially since she fought against having someone who would come by regularly to care for her and the house.

We knew that the window of time for her remaining in the house, given those conditions, was starting to close. We felt a pressure to find a solution – soon!

We knew that we didn't have many good choices, other than moving Mama to Louisville. The options for a nursing home or competency hearing we had been discussing for months didn't work for multiple reasons.

The only thing that now made sense was this new, creative plan that had seemingly come to us "out of the blue."

At some deep gut or psychic level, I knew that this strange idea to move Mama was our answer. It was the way out of our impasse.

As we discussed things, we came to an agreement that moving Mama to Louisville was the best solution for her and all of us. We knew that subterfuge was the best and kindest choice.

That wasn't an easy choice. However, it resonated with each of us as the best option. It meant we would lie like rugs and make up stories in order to reduce her risks and provide her with compassionate and safe care. It would require an interesting set of storytelling skills. Thank goodness we had been raised in the Southern tradition of storytelling. It served us well.

We began talking much more specifically with Mama about this trip and how much Tom and Ann needed her to visit. We discussed, reviewed, and tested our agreements and strategies, making sure we were all on the same page. We looked at dates. We all talked with

Mama, emphasizing how much Tom and Ann wanted and needed her to come to visit. She responded to their expressed need, which was an important learning for all of us. She needed to be needed.

To our joy, Mama became interested in making this trip to visit Tom and Ann.

We learned a very important lesson from that conversation. And the lesson is this:

All of us need to be wanted and needed. It's important for us as humans to feel that we have some worth, something to contribute, some meaning to others, especially those we love. Mother was losing a great deal, and she very much needed to be needed.

As I realized this about Mama, it reminded me of another, similar encounter years ago with Gram when she was ninety-nine years old and very frail. It was just a few months before she died. She was living with Mother and Dad full-time at this point, and I was visiting prior to a meeting of the General Assembly of the Presbyterian Church. I had mimeographed a three-page article on older adults that a group of us was presenting, and it needed to be collated. One evening, I mentioned to Gram that I might need her help collating the next day. Gram, who by this time slept until past 10 a.m., was up soon after sunrise the next morning. She came into my bedroom and woke me up with the question: "Do you want me to help you with your project?"

As we talked with Mama over the coming days, she became increasingly interested in and committed to going to spend part of the winter with Tom and Ann. Spending the winter with family was an old tradition of ours, as Gram had spent winters with us for most of my childhood and adult years. She increased her length of stay as she aged and became more frail. We began to plan for this trip of Mother's. Mama participated actively and willingly from the time that we told her that Tom and Ann needed her there with them. What a blessing and a reminder: we need to be valued and needed for our entire lives, no matter what.

For the first time in months, or years, we began to have hope that we would be able to manage her care and keep her healthy and safe.

As we talked, we further developed the plan. We knew that Mother would really not be able to return to Winston. It would be too dangerous. This "trip," in reality, was a move. We would be moving Mama from the place where she had lived for thirty years.

Ann had been looking at possible houses to purchase for some time, and, as we moved forward, we realized this was the wisest course of action. At that time, Mother's Alzheimer's was such that she was becoming impaired and not able to live alone without help, but not so impaired that she needed to be in a caregiving situation all day. As much as we loved her, we all know that, given her penchant for worry and drama, Mother would drive Ann and Tom nuts if she lived with them. And Tom and Ann would drive her to distraction.

Ann, the enterprising real estate agent, had already found a number of options. Luckily, she was able to locate a house with a layout much like Mama's a few blocks away from where they lived that wasn't terribly expensive.

Luck, grace. It was a gift, in any case. We arranged to buy the house for Mama and plan for her trip to Louisville.

We now had a clear plan for moving Mama.

Over time, we became engaged in spinning the yarn, and it helped as we grew to half believing what we shared. Ann managed all of the real estate tasks and the closing. Even though the house was just a few blocks away from their home. We knew that acclimating Mother to a new *home* would be difficult at best. However, the place was very close to Tom and Ann, and had a layout that wasn't terribly different from Mama's place in Winston-Salem.

Though it didn't have the yard lot full of azaleas, we planted many new azaleas for her that spring after we moved her.

Reflection: Balancing Independence and Supportive Care

We were very lucky that we had the option of buying a house near Tom and Ann. I realize that many families don't have the luxury of purchasing another property for a parent to move into and live close to one of the children. In fact, a parent's home is often sold in order to pay increasing expenses incurred in caregiving. Those expenses have only increased in cost in the years since Mama died. It's expensive and it's difficult to manage all of the pieces.

More elderly and their adult children are looking to reverse mortgages to fund the increasing costs for caregiving. A dear friend of mine, Jody, did that about five years ago, and the reverse mortgage was a lifeline. She had a number of us who helped out, including a friend who was a financial wizard, and an attorney. There are many different kinds of reverse mortgages that can strip down the value of the house and the payout, so careful research is critical to success.

Some families may sell property in order for their loved one to move in with one of the family members, a smaller home, a retirement community, or assisted living. Even though one's assets may not be what Mother's were at that time, many older people now in their seventies, eighties, and nineties have resources or benefits available. Many of today's elderly are often more forward-thinking, flexible, and resourceful than my mother was.

In caregiving, each of us will find that we and our loved one struggling with dementia have unique needs, challenges, resources, and assets. It is when we can bring our resources and assets to address our needs and challenges that we can move forward. Some of our answers come from research, other ones appear as creative impulses, and ideas "out of the blue."

In our case, we had two big challenges: (1) Mother's fast declining health and memory, and (2) her absolute unwillingness to consider options and her rages and unstable behavior when she felt cornered. Mama had become a real risk to herself. She was no longer able to cope alone. That was the biggest challenge. We were clear in our belief that her overarching need was to be able to live as independently as possible with help, so that she would be protected and safe, and able to continue to enjoy her music and things she still loved.

Our resources included the four of us, her other family and friends, her financial resources, and our commitment to working to find good and meaningful solutions. Every one of us caring for a loved one with Alzheimer's has a different set of skills and challenges. Find your islands of excellence, your resources, challenges, boundaries, and passion points. Develop clarity about those passion points: what you most want to do, have skill for, and can do. Then, do the best you can with what you have.

We are all very grateful that Mother and Dad were such savers and had the financial assets they did. Because Mama was a real mess and needed a lot of what had been saved to pay for her care. If we had not had the financial assets that were available, caregiving would have been so much more difficult. Our country needs to develop many of the resources for elders that we find in many European countries.

We all have resources, they just vary. One of your most challenging and life-affirming tasks is to research and go deep to find resources and assets to address the very real and often overwhelming needs and challenges.

Do an inventory. Go to those websites and local resources that have provided help to you in the past, and look for more formal and informal resources. Look carefully at your options. Talk with people who have been through a similar situation to yours.

If your biggest challenges are finding affordable or subsidized caregiving for the workday, then look for people who have solved that problem.

If you need to find inexpensive ways to remodel a part of your house to add a bathroom to the room where you plan to move your loved one, find people who have done something similar.

The local or state Alzheimer's Association and your local Senior Center can often provide you with invaluable free information and counsel. Faith communities and area nonprofits may be helpful resources as well, and can point you to other resources.

Chapter 10: Taking Care of Ourselves

Taking care of Mama was a real challenge. It was hard to know what to do. Even though I have a background in social work and health care consulting, it was still so hard. That's the way it is when you're dealing with a family member who is struggling with their own frailty and in need of a lot of support. When Alzheimer's is an issue, it simply complicates everything. She didn't realize that she was not able to care for herself when that time came.

To say that it was stressful for all of us is an understatement. Ann and Tom provided day-to-day care and managed her care in Louisville for almost two years. When it was time to move Mama again from Louisville, KY, to Buffalo, WY, the two of them were exhausted. Absolutely wrung out. But then, I'm getting ahead of myself again.

And we were lucky. We had family members willing to spend time with Mama and work to manage her care. And we had some financial resources that allowed us to hire people to share the burden. Without those resources, I cannot imagine how we would have managed.

It was a burden we willingly shouldered. We loved Mama and wanted to make sure that she received the same kind of care at home that she had given her mother. But make no mistake, the caregiving was a burden. A burden that fell primarily upon Tom, Ann, and John.

We thought that we went into these decisions with our "eyes wide open." For the most part we did, but more intellectually than emotionally. My brothers and I are all three researchers, and that skill was invaluable to us. We researched so many aspects of Alzheimer's. We studied the different care options available, and what to expect.

Even as well-equipped as we were, there were so many surprises. The journey itself was stressful, exhausting, beautiful, and sacred. All of those things. It was most stressful and exhausting on the emotional level. It was most liberating and uplifting on the spiritual level.

We saw our mother diminish over time. She grew smaller and thinner over the final years of her life until she was quite thin and frail. Mama's mind became foggy, and she leaned on her social skills. As Alzheimer's took over her brain, much like the Alabama kudzu covers the hillside, we saw her continually stumble to express herself. Her efforts at socializing at the end were painful to watch.

Music was Mother's dear friend throughout the entire ordeal. It gave her joy and pleasure and filled her life with meaning long after her mental faculties had become seriously compromised.

Her spirit was strong for most of that journey. She was usually headstrong, often controlling, and very strong-willed. It made caregiving sometimes difficult. And it also enabled her to soldier on with greater strength and dignity than had she caved in or given up at an earlier stage, or had a different personality type.

She also had a deep faith that carried her. We all read some of her oldest and dearest-loved Bible stories and reflections. The 23rd Psalm carried her a long way.

To see all of that in its very real presence was difficult. It was extremely stressful for all of us. There were enough times when I vegged out in front of the TV with my favorite chocolate. Or ate too much. There were times I disappeared addictively into work. Most of those responses and others, like drinking or gambling, are all unhealthy ways we blow off steam. I exercised many of the unhealthy options, as most of us do from time to time.

What really gave me life, and what really helped me, were the healthy stress reducers.

What are some of the healthy stress reducers that worked for me?

Prayer, meditation, support from friends, time in nature, and exercise.

Rooted in both the Christian faith, as a Presbyterian, that set of beliefs has stood me in good stead. I believe in God, and in the teachings that

Jesus left us for living. The hope of faith is a blessing, and a treasured gift.

Since the late 1990s, I have been practicing Vipassana Buddhist mindfulness practice and meditation. That has been a godsend. I tried to meditate some every day, even if it was for a few minutes. I would sit and try to clear my mind. We have a number of meditating communities in Santa Fe, and I took advantage of group meditation as well. Today, we have even more resources than I had in the late 1990s, including wonderful meditation books, downloads, and communities. What meditation did for me was to still my racing mind, and to help me realize that life is impermanent. The joys and sorrow are temporary. It provided some distance and perspective and calmed me.

I'm a rather fast-paced Gemini, so calming me was a really good thing for me and those around me!

Prayer is a wonderful practice that feeds the heart and soul. I prayed a lot. Those "Oh God, if you just do this one thing" kind of foxhole prayers, as well as regular prayers that Mother and all of us be supported and led in what we were to do. I asked friends to pray for us. I have always believed in prayer. It's just not a straight-line I-ask-God-gives kind of deal, but more like particle field theory. We share our prayers and they go into this great cosmic field. That's what I believe anyway. It was fascinating to discover that Harvard researchers were able to scientifically document the efficacy of prayer. It helped knowing that we were praying and that people were praying for us. How prayers are answered, that's for God to know, I certainly can't figure it out.

As we continued providing care for Mama, we began to encourage one another to take time off and to take time out. We encouraged each other to look at little opportunities to relax and rejuvenate. I recommend that to anyone who is a caregiver for a loved one with Alzheimer's or another form of dementia. Look for ways to feed your mind, body, spirit, and soul. What each of us needs is particular to us as an individual. One person's tonic is another one's toxin. But, when we give ourselves healthy little gifts throughout the weeks and months, it makes the journey so much easier.

"It is a marathon and not a sprint," Gloria Steinem said about the feminist movement back in the 1970s. It also applies so well to caregiving. Pace yourself. Try to realize early on that you won't get everything right. You won't get a lot of things right. However, if you get the big things right, you're doing wonderfully. Wonderfully, indeed.

Reflection: Resources for Mindfulness and Self-Care

Each of us has our own unique personality, skills, and needs. Take an inventory of yourself to help you determine what might best help you to reduce stress:

1. *What can you give, and how do you want to provide help?*

2. *What do you find difficult to do, that you'd like for someone else to handle? Perhaps another family member, friend, or neighbor can handle some of those things. Or some may have to be more limited or go by the wayside.*

3. *What do you need to recharge your batteries? What gives you food for your soul? It could be a walk outside, spending time with a grandchild, or some special project that nurtures you. Find ways to take blocks of time to feed your soul – an afternoon, or a day. Whatever you can manage. Then, find little tiny slices of time where you can nurture yourself. A fifteen-minute stroll over your lunch break, a night of karaoke, paddling on the river, or a quiet moment in prayer. It's whatever fits for you.*

Self-care is so important for all caregivers. We often find that we become sick as a result of caregiving. It can certainly age us. Mother had taken care of Dad during his final years battling cancer. After he died, we realized she had aged a great deal, and she became ill.

Take care of yourself. Look at ways you can reduce your stress. Nurture yourself. Take time for yourself. Even when it feels like you don't have a minute to spare, do things that feed your spirit.

Chapter 11: Packing and the Farewell Party

Once we had our plans for moving Mama, things moved along well. Thank goodness! It had been a very stressful few years, for the most part. It was such a relief and felt nice to come upon an easy patch. Friends of hers came forward, and we planned a number of parties for her. We wanted her to spend time with friends, and experience what they had to share about what she and her work meant to them.

We had a bit of experience with the party business. The year before, we had held a retirement party for Mama. It had been clear then that she was no longer able to manage her three remaining music students, and we felt she needed some help to retire. We didn't want her to find that her last few students petered away, with no recognition of her work and her contributions.

The retirement party started out as a simple and small affair at home with current and former piano students, during what was to be her next to last Christmas in Winston-Salem. We worked with a few of the families she had taught for years to plan a party. John, the youngest, knew many of the families and worked to contact them. It was amazing how many people were interested in coming to pay their regards and their respects.

Mama was an excellent piano teacher, focusing on the unique talents, needs, and issues of each student. She would spend hours at the music store poring over pieces she thought each student would find challenging and interesting. No student was ever turned away for lack of funds, and she provided scholarships where needed. My brother, John, who is a wonderful pianist, teacher, and composer, has carried on that great tradition.

About twenty-five or thirty people showed up for an afternoon where we feted Mama. She loved it. A few of her former students made presentations and comments. Many brought food. We had a silver tray engraved and provided her with that, along with a host of other "goodies." It was a wonderful event that surpassed our expectations. She had given a lot to the community, and people were happy to share their thanks and best wishes.

We wanted something like that for her as we planned to move her. We worked with her friends at the church to schedule a party for her after church the Sunday after Christmas. Her friends knew that this was a goodbye, but we billed it as a "Farewell for the Winter."

This provided her and her friends with the opportunity to say "goodbye." Closure is important for all of us, and we wanted this to be possible for her and her friends, even with the challenges that accompanied her departure.

The party was a lovely affair, with many people dropping by to wish her well. As usual, Mama was somehow able to be "up" for the event. Even with what was now moderate Alzheimer's, she rose to the occasion. She greeted people and talked with everyone.

It was amazing to see how well her deeply ingrained Southern social skills helped her. When in doubt, she could fall back upon these great truisms:

> "Oh, it's so nice to see you again."
> "You look lovely."
> "Yes, I'm looking forward to this trip."
> "How are you doing these days?"
> "Thanks so much for coming."

These social skills were so deeply ingrained, they were part of her old memory that lasted long into her dementia. They were second nature to her. And they served her very, very well. Even though it may no longer be popular with some folks, learning manners and social niceties might serve you well into old age. Reading and developing a large vocabulary when you're young also helps. Synonyms are one of the great tools in the fight again Alzheimer's.

People were genuinely sad to see her go. She had been an active volunteer in the Presbyterian Church and a strong supporter. Years before, she was the President of Presbyterian Women. She had quite a few friends from those years, as well as others she had met more recently, like Louise. The room was full. It was a blessing that filled her and us.

Reflection: Dealing with the Series of Small Losses

When a loved one is struggling with Alzheimer's, we all suffer through a series of small losses. It's a terrible thing to have people, places, and memories just fade away. We all need the opportunity to grieve these losses and to have closure whenever possible.

I remember when I was serving as a chaplain at Riverview Home for the Aged in Philadelphia. There was a wonderful old man there named Bobby who people loved because he was self-effacing and funny. And he was a man in a sea of women. He was so popular. Then he died. His death almost went by without notice. Except that people told me about it, and we put together a ceremony. Some shuffled in. Some were attentive, others were in a fog. They told him they loved him. They respected his memory. It brought them peace.

Take note of these times if you can, as you go through your own journey with your parent, your partner, or other loved one. Take a few moments to acknowledge these changes in activities that fit for your own family. It's a way of honoring them and yourselves.

Chapter 12: Driving Down to Georgia

We left for Louisville by way of Georgia to give my brothers time to set things up. We headed for Tula's in Athens, Georgia, not on "The Midnight Train," but in my rental car following the church farewell party for Mama. She was on a high as we left the church, and so pleased that people had come out to wish her well as she went to Louisville "for the winter."

But like Gladys, we, too, had a one-way ticket, and Mama was not to return to Winston-Salem. From the church parking lot, we headed out of town and southward. I had packed Mama's suitcases and mine the day before and my rental car was loaded and ready for the trip.

For a while, Mama didn't notice we were driving on the interstate, away from Winston. However, after we had chatted about the party for over a half hour, she finally commented:

"When will we get home?"
And then, "This doesn't look familiar. Are we going the right way?"

Even with Alzheimer's, she had moments when she was quite sharp. They would almost invariably come at the worst possible time.

After thinking for a few minutes, I came up with some of the excuses I had worked on for the previous few days.

"Mama, we're headed down to Tula's. The weather is getting bad, and a snowstorm is coming. We had to leave from church to miss it."

"But I haven't changed. I haven't even packed."

She started to fidget, and I began to worry. She had opened a car door when the car was moving once or twice before, and I dreaded the prospect of her doing that on I-40.

"Mama, we packed yesterday, do you remember? And I have your suitcase in the trunk. We're all set."

She turned and looked at me with a withering glance, not all that unknown to me. I chatted away. Finally, we either found a radio station that played the Andrews Sisters, or I started singing "Chattanooga Choo Choo." After a while, we were both singing through our now limited repertoire of WWII songs.

After that, I finally relaxed. The drive down to Athens, Georgia, was only about five or six hours, and a nice, easy trip most of the time. My nerves dragged it out, I'm sure. But after the musical interlude, we chatted away, commenting on the landscape, music, and the upcoming visit with Tula.

Mother was looking forward to the visit once her concerns had been addressed. Tula was the second youngest sibling, six years her senior. They had always been very close, with Tula often serving as her "Little Mama." In fact, when Gram had been absorbed in art projects and music lessons, it was Tula who had made sure that Mama had a good breakfast and was dressed properly for school, and the one who made sure that her homework was finished, and school requirements met. That's why Mama called Tula her "Little Mama" when she was growing up.

Soon after dark, we arrived in Athens, tired, hungry, and ready for a break. Tula was, as always, welcoming and happy to see us. But she was showing a new level of tension. After Mother had gone to bed, Tula mentioned to me that, although she felt that we were doing the right thing for Mother, she was still a bit upset. She shared how hard it was to see her little sister struggling with dementia. It was breaking to hear. Tula was much sharper than Mama, and it was disconcerting for all of us to see how much Mother had changed and what it meant.

We visited Tula for a week. I realized later that our visit had been extremely difficult and draining for Tula. It was devastating for her to see her little sister, Lorene, who was once so full of life, articulate, and energized, now so changed. Mama was now confused, rather often inarticulate, sometimes glassy-eyed, and clearly in the grip of a mental monster.

Mother had begun to have what people often call "the Alzheimer's look." When she was tired or confused, her eyes would glass over, a vapid smile would take over her mouth, and she would appear almost childlike. Her face was beginning to change. Her vocabulary was diminishing markedly. Mother, who always paid a great deal of attention to her appearance, started to look rumpled and unkempt.

The growing difference between Mother and Tula was significant. Tula and I would both manage our conversation so that the topics were familiar to Mama, and the language simplified in order to keep her engaged. But engagement was becoming more of a challenge.

The visit was pleasant, however. Tula was incredibly helpful. More than helpful, she was absolutely key to our being able to handle the change. We did things that were fun. Music, which was always a bond between all three of us, continued to serve.

It was amazing to see how much more ably Mother behaved when either talking about music or playing the piano. Many who are experts in the field of dementia have found that those who play musical instruments and who have spent their lives steeped in music tend to not forget music in the same way they forget recent events during early and mid-stages of Alzheimer's disease.

Reflection: Managing Travel

Taking a loved one with dementia out for car rides can often be fun and allow them to enjoy the scenery. We learned that, with Mama, it might have been helpful to find out how to manage her sudden urges to get out of the car. She didn't try to do that on the trips when we were moving her. However, she did try to do that one or two other times with one of my brothers, and he was quick to respond to keep her safe!

Moving can be an exciting adventure when we imagine our new place, or after settling in. But going through the packing, moving, and unpacking can be tedious and exhausting. It's even more the case with our frail, elderly loved ones. See what you can do to chunk it down into manageable pieces and look for ways to make it easier to manage – for everyone!

Helping others deal with the sudden decline of a loved one with Alzheimer's is difficult. Tula saw Mother at least once or twice a year. However, having her there for a week, tired, confused, and clearly progressed, was difficult and painful for her. In retrospect, I wish that there had been ways we might have understood the rate of Mama's change and its potential impact on Tula, and spent time discussing that with Tula before we visited.

One of the most important things we can do when helping a loved one with Alzheimer's is to provide opportunities for them to listen to their favorite music, to sing songs they love. If they play a musical instrument, see if they can try to keep a hand in playing what they can. Music enlivens people and helps them connect with life.

Chapter 13: Difficult Family Relationships

It took me until I was well into my thirties before I realized that Mama, who we had always called "a little bit crazy," was, in reality, mentally ill. Southern women were often given latitude to be a bit eccentric, as part of one's creativity and personal drama. Southern family stories and literature are full of tales of women who were much more interesting because of the drama created around them. Mother certainly brought drama into our lives.

She was brilliant, beautiful, creative, and a marvelous teacher. She provided us with a wonderful education. She ensured that our young lives were filled with learning, culture, adventure, travel, pain, and drama. She too often lived on the edge and tried to pull us there with her as she struggled.

Initially, it was hard to admit my mother was really crazy, or mentally ill. In the South, we would often talk about a situation being crazy, or someone acting crazy. A lot of that was hyperbole for eccentricities that were acted out in the "Auntie Mame" part of a woman's personality.

The realization that she was really, really off dawned gradually. As I worked on my own issues, I saw things more clearly and accustomed myself to that reality. By my late thirties, I had done a lot of inner work with the help of therapists, and finally began to see through the swaddling of denial I had been wrapped in for so long.

Mama had given me many wonderful things. These gifts she provided were quite substantial. I had studied violin at the Conservatorio de Musica de Puerto Rico with one of the great Figueroas, "Pepito," and gone to the Casals Music Festivals. I went on lots of trips and experienced the cultures of many countries by living in and visiting them. Mother and Dad valued education, and I knew from an early age that I would go to college and perhaps graduate school. We traveled so much as a family. That created an internal set-point for me to continue traveling, which I love.

But Mama also provided me, and all of us, with the very difficult legacy of her mental illness. It may have been roughly equivalent in import to her positive legacy. The twin drivers of her inner demons and the force of her personality when facing challenges were, for many years, rather overwhelming.

Like other adult children, my brothers and I tried to ferret out the cause of Mother's craziness, and had many discussions about the issue. Her father, a brilliant doctor who graduated from Vanderbilt Medical School at age twenty-three, had lost very few patients and had helped to build one of the great hospitals in Birmingham.

According to family legend, he initially drank when he would lose a patient. But eventually, he probably drank to drink. His brilliance came with an extremely volatile personality and a temper that became infamous. Gram was as calm and unperturbed as Grandfather was temperamental. We often said that Mother took after her father, and that her older sister, Tula, took after Gram.

We believed that at least some of Mother's emotional instability came from her genetic predisposition, or nature. A lot may have come from her life experiences, or nurture. It's hard to be sure about those things. We can only watch, learn, and work through our own issues to build greater health and well-being.

I learned after I was grown that Gram had always kept a suitcase packed for herself and Mama when Mother was a child. As his alcoholism progressed, Grandfather would increasingly fly into rages. Sometimes, he would break the furniture, and Gram would quickly shepherd the children out of the house and to a friend's or to the Y.

The stress of living this way is hard to imagine. Harder still to imagine would be Mother's ambivalence about her father. When she was five years old, she suffered a burst appendix. He performed an emergency appendectomy and saved her life. In the early 1920s, few children lived through a ruptured appendix. So, the father who created chaos and havoc in her later childhood was the same father who had saved her life in what was a celebrated surgical success.

Even though Mother glamorized her experiences in World War II, and in many ways saw them as the highlight of her life, the war must have been extremely frightening and stressful. After all, she was on the island of Tinian, where there was a lot of action, including the plane that dropped the bomb on Hiroshima. Her experience was much more than what she shared about the series of parties, musicals and skits for the enlisted men, dates with officers, and exciting travel.

As part of historical research for a thesis, my brother, John, discovered that many of the Red Cross women helped GIs write their last letters home. They were part of the terrible medical triage that occurred after battle. They ministered to those who were placed in the "too sick to survive" and the "very ill and waiting for surgery or treatment" categories. Mother also saw the crew of the Enola Gay take off and return after the atomic bombing run to Hiroshima. Her only comment was that the crew returned "shell shocked," and that they were "quickly escorted away for debriefing."

After she married, she and the family moved with Dad every few years with each new Red Cross assignment. Although she tried to make the best of things by building music and travel into our experiences, the frequent moves must have been stressful for her. In retrospect, I realize that, in spite of the wonderful cultural experiences that travel afforded, it provided little stability or a home anchor. Gram was the anchor – for all of us.

The moves continued. We relocated to Puerto Rico in 1963 from Montgomery, Alabama. For me, the multi-racial environment was a lifesaver. Puerto Rico was more difficult for Mother because her support network was removed. She suffered greater stress, and her behavior became more erratic. Even though she had what she called "knock-down-drag-out-fights" before we moved to Puerto Rico, the episodes increased after our move. Mother would frequently fly into rages, scream and lash out at me or my brothers.

At this point, Mother began a long descent into episodes of mental illness punctuated by periods of brilliance and strong engagement with the community. As a young teenager, I found a number of escapes, mostly productive. These included excelling at school, scheduling after-school activities, music, and babysitting whenever I had the opportunity.

The combination of these allowed me to limit my time at home, but not enough. Mother began to have violent episodes that often (but not always) came on her like a bad thunderstorm. We could usually see or sense the first clouds and then watch as the clouds darkened along with her spirit. She would become increasingly agitated and looking for a fight.

During our teen years, Mother continued to have these rages and fights. She was often able to maintain a public face of Southern charm and professionalism as she taught school and volunteered in the community. The understanding of child abuse was not yet developed, nor was the term used as we find today. People did not interfere. I did have a number of adult neighbors who had me babysit for them, and who more or less adopted me and encouraged me to spend time with them in their homes. I've often wondered how much the neighbors heard. When Mother was in one of her episodes, she would scream at the top of her lungs, as would we. Sometimes she would run outside screaming, too, once with a knife. It was probably not a secret. But nobody I knew mentioned that they understood the hell we all lived with. And nobody suggested that she might need help.

Like so many families with problems and secrets, we all suffered. Our relationships were a strange amalgam of care and great opportunities mixed with threats and violence. We learned at young ages to check the temperature of the house whenever we came home. We became hyper-vigilant. We also internalized the message that we, as the children, were to blame for the family's arguments and difficulties.

After Mother finished with one of her rages, she would be exhausted and take to her bed with a "spell." Dad's role was then to minister to her and care for her as she dealt with migraines. Before we could go to bed on any such day, he would round us up and force us to apologize to our now prostrate and very ill Mother for having made her sick. Each of us would apologize in our own way, and then she would tell us that she loved us, and that tomorrow would be a better day. This created an internalized self-blaming that we carried with us for too many years.

Decades later, when Mother began to show signs of dementia, it took all of us working together to find a way to deal with her. There were us three, and Tom's wife, Ann, who was amazing. We had never gained full adult or emancipated status in Mother's eyes, even as middle-aged adults. Taking charge required concerted effort, coordination, "moxie," and therapy. In a strange paradox, it was Mother's model of caring for her own mother, Gram, at home that gave us some of our guidance and provided some calm, sacred space and hope for all of us.

Some might wonder why we didn't report the abuse, or run away, or distance ourselves further once we were adults. It was what it was.

John and I did a lot of our own work, to make peace with our childhoods, and to gain a firmer footing as adults. As children, we knew our family was troubled, but we didn't realize that we were that unusual. There were few venues in the 1950s and 1960s for lodging complaints or getting help for oneself and one's parents. I knew I fought with my mother more than did my friends, but I did not dare talk about all that happened at home. "Nice families" just didn't do that.

Gram took care of me every summer, when I would usually stay with her long after the rest of the family left to go back home. She also came to live with us in the winter. She was my favorite person in the world, and my lifeline. She was my guide, mentor, protector, and much-loved grandmother for all time.

My parents put me through college and graduate school. By the time I realized that something had been very wrong with at least part of my childhood, I was working on my own issues. I also realized that my parents had done quite well with their investments. They helped me a number of times during my twenties and thirties, and then later on began gifting each of us annually to reduce the size of their estate.

As an adult, I did not want to rock the boat and jeopardize their financial assistance and my inheritance. I felt that they owed me. The problem with that attitude was that it kept me angry, dependent, and financially dysfunctional for many years of my adult life.

Now, as someone in her seventies, looking back over the decades, I am amazed that the three of us have done as well as we have. All of us have graduate degrees: Tom with his PhD.; John with an A.B.D. PhD. (All But Dissertation), and me with an MDiv and DMin. We've all contributed to our communities and feel good about what we've done with our lives.

I believe each of us has made peace with Mother and our childhoods. She had significant handicaps, and she did the best she could with those. Today, we're all a bit more sanguine about those experiences. We appreciate what she gave us. We are saddened by the damage she inflicted. Together, we decided that we would provide her the sort of care she gave to Gram, and none of us regrets that many years later.

We spent the money that Mama and Dad saved first on her care. What was left was divided between us, along with her furnishings and art. It was a good decision for us.

Reflection: Family Issues

If you have issues with your loved one who has dementia (and most of us have), deal with them if at all possible. Work through those issues with a therapist or other trusted adviser. Support and self-help groups can also be helpful. I didn't have regrets when Mother died, and I'm very grateful for that.

Whenever possible, take care of those issues so that you can make peace with them and yourself. Making peace doesn't necessarily mean "making nice." Part of making peace for me before Mother became ill meant setting boundaries with her, and limiting time spent during visits to reduce the potential for arguments.

The inner work I'd done over the years allowed me to better understand what I could and could not do in terms of my contributions to helping Mama during her final years. That was life-giving for me. It also allowed me to be more fully present for her, to help in ways I was able to love her and set boundaries.

Dealing with my issues and making peace allowed me to accept her more easily during her final years, and to have no regrets when she died.

Chapter 14: Moving and Selling the Winston House

Once Mama was settling into the new place in Louisville, we started to talk about how to handle the now-empty house in Winston-Salem. We knew we wanted to sell it, but didn't want to just sell it out from under her. She would surprise us from time to time and talk about Winston and the house. We usually found a way to chat a bit and then change the subject.

We were concerned about the empty house, and the potential for problems with upkeep or emergencies. It was now spring, and we realized the best time to sell the house would be during the spring or summer. We began to look for a realtor in Winston, discuss the sale, look at any work that needed to be done, and pricing the house.

It is always a challenge to handle a house sale long distance, which is what most of us face as we care for elderly parents. Having a knowledgeable resource like Ann was a big help. She guided us in finding a realtor who had a high success rate, was knowledgeable, trustworthy, and a good fit. When we sell a house long distance, we depend heavily on the realtor in our loved one's hometown, and having a good relationship is extremely important.

My brother John came up with a brilliant idea for how to help Mama divest herself of the house – emotionally and actually. It was another tall tale with the best of intentions.

He and Tom talked with Mother about the house in Winston needing a number of repairs, especially to the old clay pipes that were under the large front lawn. There had been some damage to the pipes. In recent years, roots of the old trees had been seeking water, and found and entered the pipes, making them run slowly. John and Tom simply accelerated the issue and prepared a summary of high possible costs for upkeep.

We knew that Mother could never return to that house, and that its upkeep would eat into her savings. It also wasn't a good idea to keep the house vacant for too long, even though we had people checking on it and keeping up the lawn.

Tom and John and I discussed the list, and they presented it to her, sharing their concerns about the costs for the home's upkeep, which were very real.

Mama looked at the list and tossed it down on the table in disgust.

"Why don't we just sell the damn house," she said.

So, we did.

Reflection: Selling the House

Helping a parent or other loved one sell a house from a distance is a challenge at best. Each family has its own dynamics. Those often include values, attitudes, emotions, and activities that both help you move forward and gum up the works. Look at prioritizing the most important things that need to be done and have an agreement about how you plan to proceed. If possible, get that summarized in writing, to clarify expectations, and nail down the path forward.

Carefully research realtors. Study their sale statistics, and find out how well they have done with families and homes like yours. Check references and ask for the names and contact information for sales they made with homes similar to yours. Make sure that some of the references include people with homes you've chosen.

Meet with a few of your top choices for realtors and see how well you "click." That clicking thing is so important. You want to have a positive emotional connection with them, effective communication, and trust.

Involve your loved one in as much of the process as possible. Even when their thinking and decision-making is impaired, they are still present. Their moments of lucidity can come at some very interesting times. Even though we had to pretend about some things, we tried to honor her wishes, and involve her in ways that were possible.

Selling property for some loved ones and their families is already planned, and not a big deal. With others, it has been thought about, emotional, but something that is handled well. With others, there are difficulties with your loved one. There can also be differences of opinion among siblings.

Try to give yourselves time to process the emotions that come with selling the house. That can be especially helpful if it is a house that represents where you lived for many years, and has important memories for you.

Do the best that you can managing this as one of the issues you need to address in taking care of your loved one. Sometimes the sale represents a relief and brings much-needed funds for caregiving. It can be an emotional experience.

Chapter 15: When They Forget Who You Are

Mother's much-loved sister, my aunt Tula, died in the late 1990s. The family was planning her memorial service for a month or two after her death. My two brothers and I agreed that we should wait to tell Mother in person when one of us could be with her. I was planning to visit a few weeks later, so the task was delegated to me.

When I thought it was a good time to talk, I told Mama about Tula's illness and death. She took it hard, but stoically, as I thought she might. Although she didn't dwell on her death, she did remember later on that Tula had passed away. Since she had lost a lot of her short-term memory by then, it was a tribute to her relationship with her "Little Mama" that she remembered it.

My brothers and I discussed the memorial service with our cousins. Since Tula had been a violinist and music teacher, the family planned a lot of music for the service, including a string quartet. We thought that having music would be an appropriate tribute to Tula. It would make the service easier and more meaningful for the family, and would certainly be something Mother could appreciate.

Tom and Ann started talking with Mother about the service, asking her if she wanted to go. In her more lucid moments, she was quite clear about wanting to go with Tom and my sister-in-law to the service. My brother, John, and I each flew into Atlanta and drove over to Athens. Tom and Ann drove down from Louisville with Mother. We all met at our Cousin Jenny's house outside of Atlanta.

Ever the wonderful hostess, Jenny had prepared a wonderful spread of cold cuts and salads for us. It was a wonderful and emotional gathering, as some of us had not seen each other for quite a few years.

I could tell that Mother was exhausted, but my brother and sister-in-law were absolutely wiped out. They explained the ride down had been a bruising process, full of drama and arguing. Mama had been agitated and fretful, and she fussed throughout the drive down from Louisville. They were never sure if Mother was going to suddenly open a car door while the car was going seventy-five miles an hour.

She was not having a good day, which meant that nobody else was having a good day either.

Once at Jenny's house, though, Mama perked up. She always had the ability to "put on her best face," to be charming, especially in social settings. Even with her Alzheimer's, she could still socialize and fall back upon manners and social skills she had honed for decades. It was fascinating to watch and taught me a great deal.

After eating, I got up to check on something in the next room. As I came back into the dining room, I saw Mother standing quite still and watching me with her head tilted and a quizzical expression on her face.

When she saw me return, she began to walk toward me, looking confused. Then she said, "You look so familiar." All conversation ceased, time stopped, and the room was totally silent. For our talkative family, that was highly unusual.

Even though we had discussed the fact that Mother would forget who we were, we thought we were prepared. We were so not prepared! At least, we weren't emotionally prepared. I wasn't emotionally or spiritually prepared for that bombshell that meant I was no longer her daughter to her.

I was frozen in time for probably a minute or so. Then, I responded.

I don't know where my answer came from, it just came.

"That's because you've known me all my life," I said and gave her a hug.

She hugged me back and gave me a big smile, saying, "Oh, yes," confusion momentarily relieved. I felt like throwing up.

It turned out that the afternoon at Jenny's was one of Mother's high points during the trip for Tula's memorial service. That and the service itself. We were to stay at Tula's house, since it was familiar to Mother. And once there, it was strange. We were surrounded by Tula's spirit and her things, but she wasn't there. We missed her terribly.

Mama was restless and at odds with us and herself, so we tried to keep everything as simple as possible. We fixed dinner and worked to get her to go to bed. We hoped that tomorrow would be a better day.

I was in the middle of reading **Divine Secrets of the Ya Ya Sisterhood**, and stayed up late, immersed in the intertwined stories of the Ya Yas, their past, my past, and Mama's. Being very much Southern, I read it and laughed out loud. In fact, on the plane to Georgia, there were some people who gave me funny looks as I burst out laughing. It was partly the Ya Yas, and partly the joy the story provided in the relief from stress. So, yes, I read and read.

Early the next morning, we got up and had breakfast. Mama was not doing well. She was confused and full of questions. Finally, we adjourned to get dressed. My sister-in-law, Ann, came into my room a few minutes later.

"Anne, Mama needs your help. She won't let me help her get dressed. She's taken my bra, put it on over her PJs, and says she's now ready to go to church."

"Oh, brother," I muttered and followed Ann down the hall.

Sure enough, Mama was sitting on the bed, looking pleased with herself for getting dressed by herself. She had on the bra over her pajamas. A good two or three sizes too large for Mama, Ann's bra was hilariously telegraphing Mama's arrival. I tried a number of tactics, and she was just not willing to budge.

Finally, I came upon some solution I can't remember now. We got Mother dressed. Ann recovered her bra and got dressed. In a short-long while, we met the rest of the family for lunch. Afterward, we went over to the church.

First Presbyterian in Athens is a beautiful, quintessentially mainline Protestant church (minus the tall white steeple). It has a lovely Georgian-styled brick exterior and an open, sunny sanctuary. I had been many times when visiting Tula and my cousins, and always enjoyed it as much for the aesthetics as for the services.

Mama was a bit shaky but on her best behavior. She somehow knew that the service was for her sister who had died, and she was quiet and respectful. The music was beautiful, and the string quartet was a tribute to Tula and her life in music. Afterward, we took a family photo, and when I looked at it later, I could see the continuing ravages of Alzheimer's on Mama's face.

We went by Tula's house for the last time. Everyone visited, though briefly. We all needed to travel home. It had been a long, hard day.

Reflection: What to do When They Forget Your Name

One of the moments we fear the most is when a loved one forgets our name. It is a dreaded event. We may worry about it, wonder when it will happen, or hope that it won't happen. It usually does happen at some point. I have come to realize that when they forget your name and how you are associated, they may not forget everything all the time. It is still a gut punch, no matter how we frame it.

Mama, fortunately, continued to understand that we were all family of some kind throughout her illness. As her Alzheimer's progressed, she came to believe, for most of the time, that she didn't have any children. She just knew we were somehow related and connected.

There's nothing that will prepare you for the shock. It's one of the many little "goodbyes" that we face when we are caring for a loved one with Alzheimer's. Talk with others about it as part of your planning and preparation. Most people with dementia will, at some point, forget who people are, including their names and how they are related. Some remember pieces of the connection. It's painful.

Once it starts to happen, get some support. Talk with friends and family members who have been forgotten by their loved one. Work on reframing the situation so that you see it as part of their disease. Try to realize that it is not about you. It's the disease. It's one of the saddest parts of dementia, for us and for them.

Whenever you can, help them focus on what they do remember, and build those as anchors. When a dear friend of mine was going through his bout with dementia more recently, he and I planned out those anchors, or "islands of strength." We would often visit them, to help him anchor himself in what he still knew. It was calming. We would also tell stories that took him back to those places in his life that remained strong and pleasant memories. He remembered me.

Chapter 16: Tough Choices and Taking Charge

As time passed, Mama could not function without a lot of help. We now were handling all of her care, financial affairs, and the house sale. Everything. But she still had enough moments of lucidity that she would often argue with us about how things needed to be done.

After all, she was the mother and we were her children. She had a deep need to be in charge. Whenever a lucid opportunity arose, she would stubbornly assert her will. It was almost always at the most interesting and inopportune times.

She did not like to go to the doctor. When Mama was living in Louisville, it took all of Ann's persuasive skills to get her dressed, out the door, and to the doctor's office. One time, Dr. H. was running late. Very late. After about twenty to thirty minutes of waiting, Mama announced: "This is ridiculous. I'm going home."

She promptly stood up and stormed out. Ann ran to catch up with her. Mama was moving fast, and seemed to know her way out of the building and to the parking lot. Ann took her home, and they had to reschedule.

It was not easy to take charge of situations with a mother who had a desperate need for a rock-tight hold on things. But we had to do it. Sometimes gradually, when that was possible. However, Mama was losing her ability to care for herself, so there were many times when one of her children or a caregiver had to "lay down the law," as she would say.

Thank goodness she didn't try to drive anymore. Another blessing was that she didn't leave the house and wander, as some people do. But she tried to turn on the stove from time to time. She also did interesting things with appliances. We posted large signs. When that didn't work, we removed some of the appliances.

There were those times when we had to take charge and order, persuade, or cajole her to do something. Like get dressed. Or brush her teeth. Or get in the car to go somewhere, like the doctor's office.

She couldn't dress herself anymore without help from someone else, but she didn't want the help and often complained. We shopped for dresses for her that were easy to pull on and take off. We had to reduce the number of buttons or snaps or other "do-dads" as she called them. They were confusing, and made dressing more complicated and difficult for us all.

Someone who had been a fashion plate all of her life had taken to dresses that were shapeless and simple. Thank God she no longer paid much attention to her appearance, or cared. She seldom looked in the mirror anymore, whether from lack of interest or lack of will, we never knew. Everything became scaled down and simplified.

We didn't realize that she wasn't brushing her teeth anymore right away. It's one of those personal grooming habits that, for good reason, remains personal. However, on one visit, I noticed that her teeth were a mess. I tried to get her to brush them with very mixed results. We never knew if she had forgotten how to brush her teeth, or didn't want to bother, or found some element of the exercise confusing or frightening. During my visits, I could occasionally get her to brush, sometimes as I was brushing my teeth. But we ended up pretty much accepting that it would be hit or miss. That was one of the things that we let slide.

She seemed to be taking care of bathing occasionally and going to the toilet by herself. Her skills there were starting to slip as well, but not as badly. That was something we knew we would need to address in the future.

Occasionally, Mama would defer and do what we asked. However, she must have felt control and reality slipping during her moments of lucidity. She would argue with us often. That was, in part, a long-standing habit, and, in part, her battle with the inexorable progression of the disease.

She would argue or stomp out. Sometimes she would cry and become hysterical. We tried to find creative ways to get her to do things. Subterfuge became a fine art form.

Finally, there was a sea change in her behavior that was a godsend for us. As the dementia progressed, she became more mellow and a bit more pliable. She would do things we asked more easily, with less resistance and drama. Over time, she would more willingly participate in activities like eating or getting dressed.

It was a mixed blessing.

Reflection: When to Take Charge

Taking charge was hard for us. I think it's hard for most adult children. The roles are reversed, and until we have some practice with being the parent to our parent, it's uncomfortable. In our case, uncomfortable was an understatement. It was just tough.

Personal care is one of those items I'd never talked much to anyone about after I was ten years old or so. It was one's personal business. I would notice when someone was disheveled, or dirty, or poorly put together. Seldom did I hear much discussion about personal care except in the most summary and rather clinical fashion when older adult serving agencies would describe their services.

"We provide caregiving, which includes offering companionship, assistance with tasks around the house, personal care, and support."

That sounds rather innocuous. But, for those of us who have now provided personal care to a frail elderly person, it is a far cry from that! It can be confusing, complicated, and difficult for the adult child as well as the parent. If you're able to read about this, or talk with professional caregivers, that might provide you with a great deal of help.

Over the last few years of Mother's life, we consulted with her caregivers for their advice about how to handle these caregiving tasks. In retrospect, I realize that we didn't consult on these private details enough. We researched many areas related to Mama's care, but not much in this area.

Some of our values, attitudes, and habits are ingrained early on. We learned from Mama and Gram not to talk about personal care issues, hygiene, the body, the toilet, sex, or anything else related to those topics. My grandmother was born in 1882 and had Victorian and

Edwardian values and extremely conservative habits. Those were passed down through the generations, from Gram to her daughters, and from Mama to me. It's not discussed. That's that. Most people now are not that rigid, which is a blessing.

It would have been helpful to talk with caregivers and research things like how you get a frail elder with dementia to bathe, brush their teeth, go to the toilet, get dressed, and eat. It's also useful to know how people often step into those activities, getting more intimately involved in those very private personal care activities.

There is a time when you have to move from helping to doing, like bathing them or changing a diaper. Many of us need very practical directions for how to do this safely, with a minimum of fuss.

No matter what your family culture and tradition, one can find it to be difficult and embarrassing to be in the position of dressing or undressing one's parent or other loved one, or giving a bath, or helping them to go to the toilet. It may be both easier and more painful when caring for a spouse.

We learned from our caregivers to try to keep things as simple as possible. We realized that it helped to keep things calm, respectful, and matter of fact. Be gentle and patient, remembering that most of us will be in that same situation one of these days. Some people find that having caregivers handle these personal care tasks is one of the most helpful things they can do. If that's your situation, I would encourage you to get all the support you can in that area.

If you find that you need to handle many of these tasks yourself, talk with others who have helped a parent or loved one. Talk with professional caregivers. And look on national caregiving websites to find out recommended ways to handle personal care.

Chapter 17: Stories and Playacting

Southerners love stories. Lots of cultures have had storytelling as an important part of collective life. I always realized that story was a big part of my history and culture. But it wasn't until I started working on this book that I realized that story is deeply rooted in me, and in Mama's side of the family.

Gram used to tell stories about what it was like to grow up in the late 1880s, before the turn of the last century. She'd talk about taking the train from home to Athens, where she went to school and college. She would write home for hair ribbons and art supplies. Her husband-to-be met her during her senior year, and he "came courting." In her storytelling to me about that time, she would often break into the song "Froggie came a courtin' and he did ride, ah ha."

She would laugh as she talked about her aborted attempts to learn to drive. Dr. Whorton had a Model T Ford, and she lost control of it. The car run down a little hill, tipped over, and she got out. Dusting herself off, she informed her husband that he would simply have to drive her or she would take the streetcar. That's what she did for her entire life. She became an ace at navigating Birmingham on the streetcar that ran on tracks, powered by an electric cable (the precursor to the bus).

Gram's memories of her long history were shared with us through years of family stories. She told tales about growing up in north Alabama, and her father, the Judge, who admonished her to not eat so many sweets. She talked about the early days when Dr. Whorton was developing his practice, and about her art exhibitions. She would often share the stories behind her paintings of Jefferson Davis, Stonewall Jackson, and Speaker Bankhead – as well as her paintings of each of her children. She would talk about how she and Aunt Blanche (her best friend for seventy years) would get in trouble in school, and how they helped each other as young mothers with their children. Stories were a central part of growing up under her tutelage.

When we were children, we spent part of each summer at Gram's. After dinner, the grownups would all go into the living room to visit. Most summers, we had Sister (who lived up the hill), and Tula – and all the cousins. Uncle Bill would often come up from South Alabama, where he and his family lived. Once the adults were in the living room catching up, we children would shut the dining room door. We'd then pull the dining room tablecloth back down, so that it became our tent. So transformed, we'd enter the tent to hear Jenny's newest ghost stories. She would keep us spellbound for hours, making them up as she went along. Our cousin Palmer was her sidekick and made the sound effects. I can still remember some of the gorier stories, and the scraping sound of the old blind boatman, with the flickering light of the boat, as it made its way with its human cargo down some hidden underground culvert.

My cousin Margaret also shared stories of a very different kind. She was much older, and almost grown by the time I was old enough to read what we now call graphic novels. Margaret had a stash of some of the best, like *Mad*, *Cracked*, and the best of the comics. Both her advanced age (her late teens) as well as her willingness to share her cool stash made her the envy and the model for us younger cousins. When Gram had a houseful of family, it was just the older cousins who had the privilege of going up the hill with Sister at the end of the evening to spend the night with her, Margaret, and the comic books. I was one of the lucky ones, along with Jenny and Carolyn. My brothers stayed down at Gram's. Sister also shared stories, as well as lots of wonderful junk food. We loved them both, and her, for being our own "Auntie Mame."

Mama and Gram often told the story about how Mama contracted appendicitis when she was about five years old. They told stories about growing up with a doctor in the family, with some of the tales actually memorialized in the history of Norwood/Carraway Hospital in Birmingham. They didn't tell the other stories, about how Grandfather's world was overcome with alcohol, or Grandmother's struggles during the Depression. Those were seldom mentioned, and when shared, were often told in whispers – as if the ghosts had ears.

It came as no surprise that Mama also liked to tell stories, and could weave a great one along with the best of them. Some of her favorite stories were about her experiences in Guam and Tinian during WWII. There were stories about the performances they produced for the soldiers and sailors assigned there during the war. She talked often about the other Red Cross women with whom she had shared so much, who remained friends for the rest of their lives. She laughingly shared antics of the "Red Cross Girls."

Often, her stories about Guam and Tinian sounded more like summer camp tales than WWII in the Pacific theater. However, from time to time, when she was in a serious or reflective mood, she would let us in on just a little of the pathos and the loss that were part of her life there. We realized as adults that she had seen a great deal of suffering and death, with many of the shows and songs serving as a way to help them all get through it.

Mama told stories about her trip with Gram to New York City, when Gram went to Columbia for an art class or workshop in the early 1930s. The pictures of the two of them there "doing the town" are funny and whimsical. They clearly had a great time. That story helped us so much later, when Mama had "Sundowner's."

Mother would tell us stories about the difficult and frighteningly cold winter of 1955–1956, when she and Dad moved us from Chambley to Metz France. We moved in the middle of one of the worst ice storms on record. The pipes froze. It was almost impossible to drive. It was dark and sleeting for most of the time they managed the move.

Perhaps our history of storytelling as a family helped us to move Mama and take care of her. As we developed care for her, we found ourselves telling her stories that would help her make sense of things that were confusing. We told stories to get her to do things, like move from Winston-Salem. And we told stories to try to get her to eat, wear adult diapers, and take baths. Over time, we became engrossed in these stories and started to live in them, whether they were true, partially true, or total fabrications.

Reflection: Habits That Help Us

For many of us, there are things about our families and our culture that can help us navigate the difficult journey together into and through dementia. Whether these are songs you have sung together, family traditions, pictures, places you have visited, or deeply ingrained cultural or religious practices, they may provide you with surprising grace.

Sometimes, eating long-loved food, singing a favorite tune, or being in a certain place can bring a sense of calm and competence to one with dementia, as they feel the familiar and find themselves comforted.

If you or others have a feeling about wanting to do something, or lean on some part of your tradition, lean into that. There is probably that intuitive or spiritual part of you that can lead you toward the sort of bedrock that remains known to your loved one, even when much of the short-term memory is gone.

We went with whatever it seemed fit and worked at the time.

Chapter 18: Getting Help Around the House

Within a few months after Mother's move to Louisville, Tom and Ann realized that she needed more help at home than they could provide on a daily basis. Mama was declining rapidly and needed help preparing meals and just getting through the day. The two of them spent hours each day in caregiving, but there were gaps that needed to be filled.

Initially, Tom talked with Mama about getting a housekeeper. Her response was, by now, predictable. She didn't want one. She didn't need one. She felt she couldn't afford one. Even after multiple discussions, she would not be convinced. They pushed the point, and she pushed back.

Even though Mama was having more memory problems, she could still rise to the occasion, though not as dramatically and splendidly as before. She could be a force and command attention, especially when it involved an intrusion into her world. She was adamant, still somewhat articulate from time to time, and difficult.

Finally, either Ann or Tom must have remembered the conversations that were so effective in getting Mama to agree to come to Louisville in the first place, and they began to make headway. They talked with her about this friend of theirs who really needed Mama's help. Robbie was a young widow whose husband had died a few years before of a brain tumor. She had been through a very difficult time. She did need to find more work and would benefit from another part-time housekeeping/caregiving job.

Finally, Mother relented in order to help Tom's friend, Robbie. Thank goodness.

Robbie began her work ostensibly as a housekeeper, as far as Mother was concerned. But she was really Mama's first hired caregiver. She did take care of the house. She also cared for Mama in a wonderful way. She fixed meals and took Mama for rides. A "tough cookie,"

Robbie could cut through a lot of Mama's defenses, arguments, and posturing. This was wonderful for all of us, especially Tom and Ann. Robbie was the first person who took absolutely no guff from our mother. We learned a lot from her.

Gradually, Mama accepted Robbie, and came to count on her for help around the house, fixing meals, caring for the cat, going grocery shopping, going to doctor's appointments, and heading out for drives and ice cream. It worked well. Mama came to love her and consider her a good friend.

We all felt like we were on our way. We were, for a while.

Being close to one of her children allowed for much better caregiving and closer supervision and support. Because she was not living with Tom and Ann, the pressures were reduced somewhat. Being able to hire support made a huge difference. For the first year or so, Mama was in good shape.

Whenever John or I would visit during the first year, we would help her to plant azaleas. Mother loved her azaleas. She and Dad had planted at least a hundred azaleas in Winston-Salem, and she missed them. Within a short time, there were about a few dozen azaleas covering parts of the front, back, and side yard.

Reflection: Pacing Ourselves Through the Ups and Downs

Alzheimer's is a sneaky disease, full of shifting ground. It never gets quite solid beneath your feet. There are ups and downs with good and bad days. There are times when a loved one will hit a plateau, where there aren't the usual ups, downs, changes, and dramas. Things may seem more consistent. Your loved one may appear to be doing rather well. This is what happened during Mama's first year in Louisville, after we hired Robbie to help with her care.

We need to watch out for those plateaus, and use them for resting and building the energy and fortitude needed for the next phase. The plateaus can lure us into a false sense of stability because, during those times, ups and downs even out a bit. Things can start to hum along and seem to be more easily managed.

Enjoy the plateaus. They offer a chance for you as the caregiver to recuperate and enjoy time with your loved ones. The plateaus end, and a new stage begins where there are more memory losses and greater challenges.

To understand these stages, and the plateaus, read some of the books and visit elder care resource websites that are recommended at the end of this book.

Chapter 19: The Magic of Music

"You know, Mother has almost stopped reading," Tom shared with me at our next visit, which was right before Christmas, about a year after moving Mama. "You're kidding," was my response. "Oh, she still has the *Daily Word* by her bed, but she isn't reading. I haven't seen her with a book in weeks, perhaps months." He looked at me and shook his head.

We were a reading family. When I was growing up, we would read all the time during our summers spent at Gram's. She had bookcases all over the house. She had the old ones with the glass doors that slide up and back in above the shelf. She had the dark old open-faced tall oak shelves at the top of the stairs that had Grandfather Whorton's medical library, Mother's old McGuffey's Readers, and countless other books. There were also the small bookcases in the bedroom where I stayed. They held the 1882 *Cyclopedias* (precursor to the encyclopedia). She also had early turn-of-the-century editions of *National Geographic*, which I loved. Those early National Geographic Magazines and our own life in Europe provided the many virtual and real travel experiences that created my own personal set-point that gifted me with the love of travel.

When we were growing up, we all read. We read in the afternoon in the summertime, and we read before going to sleep. Each one of us always had multiple books piled on our bedside tables. Mother loved books.

"She's really at a loss." Tom shook his head. "She wanders around a bit more now. Since she's not reading, she doesn't have much to entertain her other than the piano. She does play the piano a lot, which is good."
"What about television?" I asked.

Tom explained that she couldn't follow many of her favorite shows anymore, like "Murder She Wrote." The plots were too complex. She would ask a lot of questions when Ann and Tom watched TV with her. When she couldn't understand what was going on, she would say that the stories were silly and stupid, and she would often get up in a huff and turn off the TV, much to their frustration if they were engaged in the plot at the time.

John was coming soon, so the three of us would have a chance to talk and look at options. We discussed the problem. This was tough. Mother and all of us got so much joy from reading that I couldn't fathom not being able to read. Or finding it too confusing.

This was just one of many of her losses.

It was John's idea to go to the video store and look for movies that we thought she knew, and would like. We did that, hopeful that we would find something. We tried one or two, and they were dismal failures, real bombs.

Finally, we happened upon *The Sound of Music*. She had taken us to the premiere in 1964 when it first came out. We went to this large movie theater in San Juan. It was such a long show that it had an intermission. We all loved it. At least, I remember that Mother and I did.

When we played the video, we were mildly hopeful. What a pleasant surprise to find that she not only loved it, she was more engaged than we'd seen her in months. We tried it the next day, and she loved it again.

This is another example of how we found a solution by happenstance, through trial and error. Someone had a creative idea, and we worked with it. We kept trying things. What finally worked was born in a creative moment, tried, tested, and built out as part of a new strategy in her care. We had found another discovery that worked. That was after testing out a number of options.

What we didn't know then was that she would watch *The Sound of Music* almost daily (sometimes twice a day) for the remaining few years of her life. It nourished her in a way that was magical.

When the movie started with Julie Andrews singing in the meadow, Mother would always say "Oh, look," or "Isn't that pretty." A big smile would come across her face. She would laugh and clap her hands. From that moment that Julie Andrews spun around in the high mountain meadow until the time that the Germans came to hunt down the Von Trapp family, Mama would watch, fully engaged, excited and alive. We discovered that Mama followed the story and enjoyed things up until the time that the Gestapo were hunting the Von Trapps and they escaped. That part of the movie frightened and confused her. We always ended the movie before that section and found a good stopping point we always used.

Little did we realize the role that *The Sound of Music* would play in our lives when it came out in the 1960s, or even after we rediscovered it for Mother that Christmas. But that movie would become one of her mainstays – and ours. Every afternoon for about two years, whoever was caring for her would get her situated in front of the television and put on *The Sound of Music*.

Each time she watched; it would be new. The story, the pictures and the music gave her many happy hours during those final years. She was actively engaged, and life had meaning, though that meaning was inexplicable to us. It was important enough to see that she would smile, clap her hands, and enter into a world that gave her great joy. When all was said and done, my brother John and I had memorized all of the songs and a great deal of the dialogue.

Reflection: Creative Solutions

Isn't it funny, the things we discover that work? When we realized that The Sound of Music *would be such a help to Mama, we were pleased, surprised, and fascinated. As she moved inexorably into the dimness of dementia, we were humbled by the process of discovering little things that gave her joy and enlivened her. The little things that engaged her. Those that helped her, and us, to cope.*

These were the little and very important things that made for a better day. We learned that one should just be open to ideas and become as creative as possible.

So, try a lot of things. It was surprising to see what works. Again, each family is different, and each person is different. What clicked for my mother will not necessarily click for your loved one. However, my experience does tell me that the human spirit is strong and resilient. Even with the dimness caused by dementia, there are sparks of life and light. And when one finds a way to connect with one of those sparks, magic happens for all of us.

I strongly recommend the movie The Notebook, *with James Garner and Gena Rowlands. It's the story of a couple who fell in love decades ago during and after World War II. The wife is now struggling with Alzheimer's, and her husband is caring for her. She goes in and out of dementia. Over time, her husband has learned how to walk with her through the ups and downs of her journey. He reads stories about their earlier life, which give her a great deal of satisfaction and joy. Those stories occasionally serve to spark her recollections, and her ability to reconnect with her husband and her life. For just a little while.*

Chapter 20: Friskies and Milk for Breakfast

Mother had been living in her new house near Tom and Ann for over a year. After her plateau, she was now beginning to lose her ability to manage many other aspects of her life. For years, she had depended upon children, caregivers, and friends for help with rides, grocery shopping, going to church, and doctors' appointments.

Early on, before moving her to Louisville, she had needed help with many aspects of her life, especially with maintaining the house, paying bills, and handling her affairs. However, after moving her to Louisville, she needed to rely on family and caregivers for much more, including cooking and eating her main meals, getting up in the morning, and getting to bed at night. She needed help with dressing as well. We found that when she tried to dress herself, she usually chose the clothes we had bought that were easy to put on, with no buttons or difficult openings.

She no longer read, although she continued to keep her *Daily Word* on the nightstand by her bed. It was an old issue, and that same monthly reflection stayed by her bedside for a long time. Someone had canceled her subscription. For a person for whom reading had been a great love, it was sad to see her no longer able to engage in one of her favorite pastimes. More than a pastime, a life-giving activity.

It was difficult to see and acknowledge the decline, probably harder for us, because she didn't seem to be that aware of the loss. Thank goodness for that. She would have been horrified.

During her first years with Alzheimer's, when she left little "sticky notes" everywhere, she was constantly frustrated when she couldn't remember things and often irate when we would correct her. However, by now, she had mellowed into some sort of gentle mental fog.

She was starting to sit for long periods with the television on, staring off into space. She could still play the piano. She knew that we were important to her, loved ones with some connection she didn't understand, but accepted.

Whereas her social skills helped her a great deal in the beginning to cover up her forgetfulness, they were now weak and tawdry props. Her smile became forced and her eyes glassy. She now almost always had that dreaded "Alzheimer's look." Whereas Mama had always walked with a purposeful stride, her gait was now much more of a shuffle.

On one of my visits to Louisville to provide some respite care to Tom and Ann, I had just finished breakfast when I was surprised to find Mother coming into the kitchen. Although she was an early riser for most of my life, she took to sleeping in during her final years.

I fixed her some oatmeal and we visited for a while. Focusing perhaps too much on tasks I was trying to accomplish, I got her settled in the den watching *The Sound of Music* and began my projects.

About mid-morning, my sister-in-law Ann came into the kitchen. She and I checked on Mother, who was still engrossed in Julie Andrews, the story, and the songs. We were so lucky to have happened upon that movie to keep her occupied. We would discover soon what a joy and a mainstay for her later on when little could grasp her attention or occupy her mind.

Ann was understandably concerned about Mother's decline. Tom came by almost every day and helped Mama with a great deal. He handled the house, helped her with meals, and he would sit with her and keep her company while he graded papers. Later on, he would often spend the night.

But it was Ann who spent hours with Mother day in and day out. I could tell she was exhausted. However, Ann never lost her sense of humor. One day, she told me about Mama's very recent experience with Friskies.

A few weeks before, Ann had dropped by to check up on Mama, visit with her, and help her with the day's activities. That particular morning, Mother was already up, dressed, and sitting at the kitchen table eating breakfast as Ann came in. She was in a good mood and offered to fix Ann some cereal and milk. Going over to the cupboard, she pulled out the box of Friskies and put it on the table. Then she got the milk from the fridge and fixed Ann a bowl. Friskies and milk.

Ann said, laughing, "I was flabbergasted. Didn't know what to do. After she fixed mine, she calmly went back to her own bowl and finished it up. I thought for a minute I'd try to stop her. But, well. She'd already started eating it before I got there. I realized that stopping her might just upset her and make things worse."

We laughed so hard we almost cried. If we hadn't been laughing, we might have cried.

But Ann was right. She wanted to protect Mother's dignity, and upset her as little as possible. She also wanted to avoid eating Friskies herself. She dillied and dallied, as we say in the South, and somehow managed to finesse the issue, dump the contents in the disposal and move Mother's attention to something else.

Reflection: Managing the Best We Can

When the decline becomes clear, we learn to manage the best we can, and prioritize things. Looking good in a matched outfit is not important if it requires difficulty dressing or a fight. If your loved one puts on plaids and stripes with a shirt that has stains from yesterday's lunch, if they can put it on by themselves, that's a little victory, and the rest doesn't matter.

You will find that the process of caregiving and walking with someone in their journey with dementia strips away many of life's "shoulds." It strips life down to its essentials, with just the bare essence remaining. It doesn't really matter if your loved one spills a drink, drops food on their clothes, watches the same show dozens of times, or puts some of their clothes on backward.

So what if your parent mixes up their memories and has stories of your childhood all jumbled up. Mama had juxtaposed our childhood home in San Juan onto the Wyoming mountains. At first, we argued. Soon, we realized that it really didn't matter.

Spending time together and finding ways to enjoy one another becomes much more important.

The decline was clear, and we did the best we could to manage the loss, the grief, and the anger. The 36-Hour Day *by Nancy Mace and Peter Rabins is what I consider to be a must-have resource. Robert Butler's "How to Care for Aging Parents," is another excellent book. Robert Butler was a friend of Maggie Kuhn's, now departed, who I met once. He seemed a very distinguished, articulate, and kind doctor to my early thirty-something self. I recently learned from a friend who knew him well that Rabins himself contracted Alzheimer's.*

These and other books and resources help us to have a better intellectual understanding of the disease and its progression. These resources provide a framework. It is often much harder to have an emotional understanding of Alzheimer's. Sharing with family, friends, and a support group help with the emotional understanding, and with acceptance.

Another resource that can be very helpful if this fits your own spiritual and religious values is mindfulness practice, whether the Buddhist or another tradition. Mindfulness teaches us that life is impermanent. If we live in the now, we can live meaningfully, joyfully, and without a great deal of pain. It's worrying about the past and catastrophizing about the future that create pain. Of course, it's easier said than done.

Each day provides its own new reckonings.

Chapter 21: Health Problems, Hospital, and Rehab

During what was to become Mother's last few months in Louisville, she became quite ill. She was increasingly frail and unable to communicate. She got a cold which became serious. Tom and Ann were watching her carefully and had increased their already significant level of caregiving.

By this time, they were providing Mama with almost 24/7 care. Robbie came most weekdays for a half-day or more. Ann spent much of every day with Mama. Tom came over in the evening to fix dinner and spend the night.

As is so often the case with the elderly, a small illness or ailment can balloon into a serious malady almost overnight. This can occur because they are not aware of what's happening, or they have a hard time communicating about the issue. Our older bodies are frailer, and what is a health nuisance to a younger person can become life-threatening to the elderly. That was the case with Mother. We later learned how much this is true as we went through our experience with COVID-19.

Within a short amount of time, Mama became very ill. Tom and Ann took her to see her doctor, and he recommended immediate hospitalization. She had pneumonia and septicemia. She was so ill that I was looking at airline flights and planning a trip.

Then, within an equally short amount of time, the hospital stabilized her. They put her on a respirator with heavy doses of medication, including IV antibiotics. Within a day, she was improving.

Being in a hospital with the noise and tubes was very frightening for her. Tom and Ann managed to spend a lot of time there, providing her with the comfort that comes from having a loved one nearby. I didn't learn until almost a decade later when I was writing this book that Mother had actually been more than a handful for the hospital staff and Ann during the five days in May of 2000 when she was in the hospital.

Mother was terrified about being in that strange and noisy place, hooked up to tubes and monitoring equipment. Afraid and unable to understand what was happening, she tried to pull off her cardiac monitoring equipment multiple times a day. She tried to pull out her IV. She did succeed in pulling out her catheter.

The physician and nursing staff talked with Ann and Tom, and said that they would have to restrain Mother unless someone was with her around the clock to ensure that she did not continue to interfere with her own treatment.

Tom was adamant that he didn't want Mother to have restraints. But he was in the middle of final exams, and could not be there more than a few hours from time to time. Ann, ever the stalwart resource, stayed with Mother for those five days. She had some respite when her own mother would come to look after things to give Ann a break.

The five days felt like forever to Mama, to Ann, and I'm sure to the staff at the hospital. Finally, after five days, Mother was stabilized. Ann was exhausted.

It was clear that Mother would recover. However, she was so frail that it was not safe for her to return home. In just a week or so, she had gone from being able to walk on her own and handle many tasks with assistance to being unable to walk, or go to the bathroom or feed herself. She needed intensive rehabilitation and was transferred to a nursing home that was also a rehab center.

Mama was transferred to a very nice private pay facility in Louisville, where she tried the patience of even the best of the nursing home staff. From the first day, Mother asked the staff repeatedly when she would be able to go home. She complained. She demanded. She pontificated. And she got better.

Once Mother was better and able to get around a bit, the nursing home staff tried to get her to play the piano they had in the day room. Mother's response was: "How can you expect me to perform with such inadequate equipment?" This comment from someone with mid-stage Alzheimer's! She was a piece of work.

After a number of weeks at the nursing home, Mama was discharged back home. A few months later, Ann decided that it might be useful to investigate nursing home care options, in case this was needed for Mother. We knew that she had now reached another level that required even more intensive care and monitoring.

Ann called a number of facilities, including that nursing home, to see what options might be available. She indicated that they had cared for Mother in the recent past.

The staff responded: "There is no availability now, nor do we see any openings for the foreseeable future."

Ann felt like they really did not want to have her come back.

Reflection: Managing the Many Health Scares

A parent's final years are often littered with health scares. These can make us think catastrophic thoughts. "This is it. This time, they won't recover." It isn't true with everyone. But many of our frail and elderly parents have a series of health challenges during their final years. These scares were an emotional roller coaster for us, and are for most families.

In today's world of managed health care, one needs to be very well-informed about options, and resources, and have a health care advocate. In most cases, adult children, a spouse, or other loved one can serve as the parent's health care advocate, to be named in the Health Care Power of Attorney, as part of the will.

As an advocate, you will want to research the different types of health care facilities that exist where your parent lives. Today, there are excellent resources online that provide ratings of doctors and hospitals. In addition, the Joint Commission provides accreditation information. Find out which hospital has the best recovery rates, the best treatment outcomes, and the lowest in-hospital infection rates. Check to see which doctors have the best ratings by patients and accreditation agencies, and which surgeons have the best surgical outcomes. All of this information is now available online. Check the resources section at the end of the book.

Discuss these issues with friends and colleagues, other family members, and people in a support group if you're part of one. It's amazing what you learn from others' experiences.

We had already developed a Health Care Power of Attorney for Mother, along with a set of Advanced Directives. We, as her children, had times we didn't feel well-equipped to handle her. However, we knew we were well-equipped with needed resources to act on her behalf. This was important, as we were able to direct her care and act as her advocates with the hospital staff. We were able to demand that certain standards of care be met, and were able to talk with staff to come to an agreement about Mother's care to avoid using restraints. If Mother's pneumonia had worsened and if she had become critically ill as she did a few years later, these documents would have enabled us to direct both her care and instruct the medical staff about what should and should not be done.

Talk with your parents about their health care wishes. If possible, do this while they are still active, perhaps as they are nearing retirement. If you have a partner, you may want to begin putting these pieces in place prior to retirement, or sooner. I have a Health Care Power of Attorney and Advanced Health Care Directives. These instruct my health care team to not engage in extraordinary measures to keep me alive just to put time in on the ventilator and add to the hospital's billing activity. Remember that the vast majority of health care expenditures occur during the final months of someone's life. I don't want to hang around to keep some accountant busy attending to the hospital's bottom line.

Do some research about the Health Care Power of Attorney and Advance Directives. If your loved one hasn't developed these yet, talk with them about creating them and providing you with copies. Ensure that you have them in place for yourself as well. Websites provide excellent information and templates. You can either use an attorney, a self-directed option, or talk with someone who works in a local nonprofit serving older adults to see what they would recommend.

Chapter 22: TSA Mishaps Mess Up Travel

We were once again moving Mama. Tom and Ann had given so much. After two years in Louisville, it was clear that Mother could no longer function at her own home, even with all of the support that Tom, Ann, and Robbie provided. The three of them had been awesome!

Mother was now much more frail and forgetful. Physically, she was weak after her bout in the hospital with septicemia and the month of rehab in the nursing home. She had moved back home, but she was more forgetful, and increasingly in a mental fog.

Even with this decline, there were times when she could be her old sharp self. She continued to play the piano. She still had the ability to understand what I was playing on the piano when I visited, and to correct me when I played something that she knew well, but with lots of mistakes. I play violin as my principal instrument, and piano just now and then. She knew almost all of my limited repertoire. It was interesting to watch her show skill in this area.

It was time to develop a new strategy that involved a lot more care. This time, the decisions were easier, partly because we had been through this before, and partly because Mother was more compliant. It was a mixed blessing, this new level of compliance.

As a group, we talked and decided that we could move Mama out to Wyoming to live with John. We had found a place in Wyoming just a few years before and had put some of the money from the sale of Mother's Winston-Salem house into the place in Wyoming, knowing that it would be a good investment regardless of what happened.

In Louisville, Ann and Tom got Mother ready to move by talking with her about her upcoming trip to the mountains, which she loved. They got her packed and ready for another adventure. John flew into Louisville to pick her up and escort her out to Wyoming.

For those people who live on the East or West coasts, it is often shocking to discover that you must spend a full day to travel from a city like Louisville to a small town nestled in the Bighorn Mountains of Wyoming. Although our planning for this move was much easier in comparison with the one two years before, we were worried about how well Mother would be able to weather this long journey.

She had been in the hospital and the nursing home just a few months before. We knew it would be exhausting for her and for John. We all tried to be both psychologically and physically prepared.

The trip started out well enough. We had a morning flight out of Louisville that was not too early for Mama to get ready and out, but not so late as to put them in Casper at midnight. There were two layovers, one in Atlanta and a second in Denver. It was grueling even during the days of the unencumbered flight. With TSA body scans, pat-downs, and questions, it was difficult at best.

In this case, it turned into an absolute nightmare.

John was able to keep Mother occupied during the early flight. The first layover in Atlanta layover was fun with lunch and talk about Atlanta. Mother still had a good recollection of the distant past, and enjoyed stories about Atlanta, which was the big nearby city when she was growing up. Like so many Southerners, we loved Atlanta as it represented both the Old South, and the new prosperity, what with Co-Cola headquartered on Peachtree Street, Delta headquartered there, and one of the largest interstate systems in the US. We did call that famous drink Co-Cola, rather than Coca-Cola, which branded us decades ago as either "true Southerners" or lazy with our speech, or both!

The flight from Atlanta to Denver was long and tiring. Mama had napped lightly, but she hadn't really slept. By the time she and John arrived at the Denver airport, she was tired, hungry, and cranky.

As airports go, Denver can often be as difficult to navigate as Atlanta. It is large, and it takes a while to get from one gate to another. Mother resisted using a wheelchair on principle, and the walks were difficult for her, even with the pedways, or mechanized "people-movers." In fact, John often avoided them because Mama became frightened by the prospect of hopping on and off of a moving belt. Whenever possible, they hopped on the little trams that took people from gate to gate, as that mode of transport was not nearly as repugnant to her as a wheelchair.

In Denver, they had to change carriers to Casper, and John was forced to go through the TSA search once again. This time, he was selected for a full body scan by TSA. Even though he explained to them that he was traveling with his frail mother with dementia, they did not appear to be either sympathetic or even interested. He was one of their chosen, and that was that.

John tried to get the TSA staff to allow him to get Mama and bring her along where she would be nearby, and watched by a TSA staffer. Mama wasn't that far away at that point, certainly within shouting distance. But they refused that request.

They whisked John away, and he felt like he was being treated almost like a criminal, while Mother sat nearby, unaware that her lifeline had been temporarily severed. They subjected John to a demeaning search, and by this point, were ignoring his pleas to watch his mother for him while he was being detained.

Impaired as she was, Mama soon noticed that John was not there. A few minutes later, a TSA staffer came running into the private screening area. "Good Lord, somebody do something. There's a crazy old lady out there screaming at the top of her lungs for Johnny. She's running up and down the aisle and nobody can calm her."

John heard that and was furious. We children learned a great deal from Mother over the years, and one of her greatest teachings was showing us (by example) how to lay into people who are both incompetent and arrogant. We do not suffer fools lightly. The bottled-up rage at the stupidity of the TSA staffers just boiled over.

"That's my mother, you idiots. I warned you that this would happen. I asked you to bring her so she could be nearby. But, no. You wouldn't listen. Well, your stupidity has just made an elderly woman sicker, and created incalculable difficulties for the final leg of our travel. You should be ashamed of yourselves. If, in the future, you find yourselves needing to care for an elderly parent as I am doing now, I hope that you're treated better than you've treated me."

They were a bit aghast at the dressing down. A few were probably ashamed, realizing that John was right, though. TSA's decision not to deal with the customer's request was a gross oversight at best, or negligence at worst. The error had serious consequences for the travelers.

Fortunately, there was someone in a supervisory position who had a little compassion and a little common sense. John was allowed to quickly get dressed, go round up Mother, and try to calm her down before they had to make the connecting flight.

He was angry, and Mother was terrified. Both were exhausted. She chattered meaninglessly for the rest of the evening, totally disoriented and dismayed. She had been abused, and so had John.

.

Reflection: Challenges of Travel

When you are caring for an elderly loved one who is severely impaired, bureaucrats can be the bane of your existence. Bureaucrats acting badly can be disruptive, harmful, or even dangerous.

How many of us have spent hours on the phone with providers who pass us on to the next person, to handle what used to be a rather simple task. It's happening for many services: phone, utility, or health insurance, to name a few. When we face problems with airline travel and TSA, hospital care or health insurance, that can hit us where are families can be deeply hurt.

Dealing with TSA at the airports can be no problem, an inconvenience, or an absolute nightmare.

How can you cope with these types of situations?

Whether it's the TSA, or a local government official, or a staffer in a health care facility, we find that many are well-trained professionals who do a good job, who have pride in their performance, and who care about those they serve. Unfortunately, there are also far too many low-level bureaucrats on the front line who provide poor service. They, themselves, are frequently caught in systems that are dysfunctional. Frontline workers often live with ineffective managers and policies that need improvement. Many struggle with poor orientation and training for their positions, low pay, and heavy workloads and add-ons to their job requirements. We have increasing challenges with workforce recruitment and retention, especially since COVID-19.

I believe that the majority try hard and do well most days. However, there are the minority who are the officious, ignorant, and arrogant staffers who can make your life a living hell, as those staffers did with Mother and John.

Your strategy really depends upon the situation. In some cases, it is possible to analyze the organization and meet with staff who are "the good ones," or to demand to see a manager. Sometimes, it is possible to demand better service or demand a change.

When possible, having two or more people meeting with the staffer will help. If you have a well-informed advocate, most staff will take pains to do a good job because they realize that their errors will not be tolerated very well. It's wonderful to have an advocate.

It's also important to document the difficulties in real time, and get the names of people that are serving you, and their supervisors, wherever possible. Then, as soon as possible, file a complaint if you feel that is safe. You also may want to report the problem to your state Office of the Attorney General or related federal or licensing oversight agency.

There will be those times when all of the best planning doesn't provide safety or protection. There are times when you don't have an advocate with you, as was true on this plane trip. During those times, if it all goes to pieces, you just do the best you can.

When the bad stuff happens (and it will), draw upon your best coping strategies. For some, it is withdrawal and silence. For others, it's a demand. For some, it leads to advocacy for oneself and others, and for others it comes out in storytelling.

We all do the best we can.

Chapter 23: Afternoon Drives in the Bighorns

Buffalo is a small town of about 4,000 people nestled at the foot of the Bighorn Mountains, near Sheridan in northeast Wyoming. Once John got Mama to the house in Buffalo, he looked for things he could do to help her settle in. One of his first ideas became a mainstay for him and for Mama. He took her out for afternoon drives in the Bighorns.

The scenery around Buffalo is stunning: large craggy peaks, high mountain meadows full of flowers in the summer, cows, cattle drives, deer, antelope, and a cobalt blue sky with a limitless horizon. He took some time in the afternoons to explore the region where the deer and the antelope really do play, along with a lot of other wildlife.

They drove through the countryside every day, usually in the afternoon. He would drive up into the nearby mountains where they would visit South Fork – not the one in Texas, but rather a horse ranch. They would drive to Ucross, a foundation and artists' colony. They would drive over to Sheridan or up into the heavily wooded tiny town of Story, with a population of a few hundred people and hundreds of thousands of beautiful pine trees.

Her eyesight and her sense of perspective were changing, and she did not realize that the mountains were many thousands of feet high and miles away. In fact, the peaks and passes are above 10,000 feet. She thought they were hills close by. I am not sure if one's ability to see or process three-dimensional viewing is lost with Alzheimer's. But her three-dimensional perspective had flattened, along with her affect and her face.

She did enjoy the drives. John varied them and pointed out scenic markers, wildlife, and cattle. Going back to old activities Mama played on long car trips with us as children, John had her count the cattle, or look for red cars. He would point out simple things like ranch houses. There was an ugly pile of used cars way out in the countryside, and, true to form, Mother always made a negative comment about it, and John used this as a way to develop conversation. He also would call out when they crossed a cattle guard in the road.

"Get ready for bumpety bump," he would say. And then: "Here's bumpety bump."

"Bumpety bump," she would respond.

It was so very basic that it almost seems silly sharing it. However, it engaged her. She was involved in conversation and interacting with John and the environment. It made her happy.

Reflection: Joy in the Little Things

As part of my work developing the book, I have thought about the kaleidoscope of experiences we had caring for Mama. I've reflected upon our decisions and their impact on all of us. And, I've considered the strange way that answers came to us.

The drives and the "bumpety bump" conversations were examples of a strategy we employed intuitively. We talked about whatever seemed to come up, and tailored our conversations to wherever she happened to be at the moment.

Over time, we were guided by the following very basic principles. They made sense and worked for us. Perhaps some will work for you.

1. Take good care of Mother, and provide her with compassionate care and companionship in her last years.
2. Keep Mama safe, clean, and dressed.
3. Provide a routine that offers reassurance.
4. Hire compassionate and competent caregivers.
5. Give her lots of small meals, with high-calorie and high-nutrition food and milkshakes to keep her from losing so much weight.
6. Develop ways to engage and occupy her (The Sound of Music, drives in the country, piano, and helping to prepare meals or set the table).
7. Engage in whatever conversation works.
8. Forget about reality-based discussions and stay with stories.
9. Look for simple ways to enjoy time with Mama.
10. Take care of ourselves.

Chapter 24: Getting Her to Eat

Like so many people who are elderly, frail, and suffer from Alzheimer's, Mama lost her appetite. She didn't have much of one to begin with, so this was a serious problem. Thin and svelte for most of her life, except during menopause, she was in the low three figures, as we were saying then. Too often, she dipped into the high two figures. Mama was just under 5′7″ and a two-figure weight represented a serious health hazard.

Again, Mama's care for Gram gave us guidance with the issue. During her mid and late nineties, Gram had pretty much lost her interest in eating. They say that we lose some of our sense of taste as we become elderly. Then, eating becomes a bit of a chore.

Mama had tried many different strategies to get Gram to eat. Like us, she experimented with lots of options. Her most successful was a high-protein, high-calorie milkshake. John used the recipe Mama developed for Gram as his base. His rediscovered milkshake included milk, chocolate ice cream (new), chocolate syrup, blackstrap molasses, protein powder (new), and part of a banana. John also added a vitamin mix. Blended in the right proportion, it tasted good and was probably close to 500 calories.

The milkshakes worked and quickly became a mainstay for Mama. By feeding her a milkshake once or twice a day, he was able to help her from losing any more weight. From time to time, she actually gained a little weight. But her weight always remained low, and it was a challenge.

Most of us become pickier with our food as we age. Our appetites are reduced, and we eat smaller portions. That's not always the case, but is often the case with women, and it was true for both Gram and Mother.

Gram loved chocolate all of her life, and one way to stack up the calories was to give her candy, ice cream, or cookies. Mama's sweet tooth wasn't as well developed as Gram's, but she did like ice cream and cookies, so those became her food staples along with the milkshakes.

Every once in a while, some well-meaning but impractical health professional would ask about her nutrition and recommend things like more green, leafy veggies. We were somewhere entirely different on Maslow's Hierarchy of Needs. We were simply trying to get her to eat enough calories to keep her going, with as much nutrition, vitamins, and protein as we could get into her. We still served her lunch and dinner, but she picked at her food, and got little nutrition from the traditional meals.

What some of these well-meaning experts didn't seem to grasp was that we were simply not able to deal with higher-order issues like green, leafy veggies. We tried to give her good-tasting, high-protein and high-calorie shakes and other food. They worked, and that's what was important to us.

Even though the shakes represented her main meals, John continued to have breakfast, lunch, and dinner at the dining room table. This was another of the important rituals that could help ground Mama and reassure her.

Sometimes Mother surprised us and would come to the table with an appetite. Those times became less frequent with the progression of her dementia and her increasing frailty. It was always a joyful occasion when she was hungry and interested in food. And that's when she would eat her green, leafy vegetables. We tried as well.

Reflection: What Happens When We Lose Our Appetites

In addition to losing our appetites as we age, we often become more isolated. Preparing and eating nutritious meals can become a hassle for us. As we become more elderly and frail, nutrition often poses a challenge. It's important to become creative and go with what works.

My Cousin Jenny mentioned that she and Carolyn had a similar challenge with their mother Tula. Her sense of taste diminished, and food no longer tasted very good. Jenny also experimented with different options, choosing those foods that her mother liked best.

Although it is ideal for one to eat nutritious, healthy meals throughout life, as we age, it becomes more important to ensure that we eat – period. We need to receive the necessary vitamins, other nutrients, protein, and calories. I'm not a nutritionist and am way out of my depth here. In fact, I like potato chips and chocolate way more than broccoli. However, many who have been involved with caregiving have shared similar experiences and decision-making processes.

There are some wonderful local resources to help both you and your parents as you look at nutrition. Senior Centers are funded by the federal government to provide nutritious midday meals. The quality and tastiness of those meals vary by location. Governmental leaders at federal and state levels realize that older adults often do not eat well. In many places, these meals provide excellent midday nutrition for a small donation. Many Senior Centers or the local Meals on Wheels also provide home-delivered meals. For those on a fixed income, these meals are an absolute godsend!

Senior Centers and local college and university continuing education departments and other nonprofits offer presentations and workshops on nutrition, nutrition and aging, and other related topics.

Chapter 25: Dr. Whorton's RX for Skin Treatments

A number of times, Mother's caregivers had tried to get her to wear adult diapers. She needed the protection, but she fought the efforts with such force that caregivers and we backed down. After she moved to Wyoming, her incontinence started to become a problem and she was damaging her favorite chair and parts of the rug.

Clean-up was a poor choice, but she still fought efforts to get her into diapers. What a mess it was. Literally.

Soon after she arrived in Wyoming, I was up visiting and witnessed the ongoing fights. When we were growing up, she and we used to call them "knock-down-drag-out fights." Only this time, our roles had reversed. The arguments were terrible. Something had to be done.

Finally, John and I had an idea. Again, it was just one of those wild ideas that "popped into our heads." By this time, we had learned to pay attention to those intuitive flashes, because they usually provided a helpful solution.

This time, we found ourselves talking about her father, Dr. Whorton. She worshipped him because, as I mentioned earlier, he had performed a lifesaving appendectomy on her burst appendix when she was a child. He was a well-known Birmingham doctor prone to rages and drink. He was both a positive and negative force in her young life, and did leave a legacy of her deep respect for his medical knowledge.

We discovered that his force still held sway for Mama.

I found myself telling another tale.

"Mama," I said. "You know that your father, Dr. Whorton, wants you to wear these special pants for your back."
"For my back?" she asked.
"Yes, Mama. He checked you out, and you need some more back support."

She gave me one of her looks, but I persevered, already deep into this wild tale.

"Mama, they will really help you. They give you support for your lower back."

I held them up to myself, pointing to the back of them, and my back. *Please, Lord. Let this one fly,* I thought.

"Oh, all right. If he said so."

"He did, Mama. He did," I said.

Mama wore her adult diapers every day from then until the day she died, without complaint, and without any further arguments.

John was especially relieved

Mama was bathing less. By this point, she was in the later stages of Alzheimer's and she really didn't notice much of anything, including bathing and dressing. She had help each morning getting dressed. Meals were now an interactive event with someone helping her to eat or drink. She watched *The Sound of Music.* And she was helped each evening to go to bed.

John and we became concerned about her personal hygiene, bathing and brushing her teeth. We didn't do very well with the tooth brushing, but we did find a way to get her to let someone give her a bath.

When we talked about having someone help her bathe, she would argue with us, stonewall us, deride us, or stomp out. Her defense mechanisms were well-honed, and she could use them until a few months before her death.

Like many women of her generation, she was extremely modest and didn't like the idea of being undressed by a caregiver. She was probably afraid of water by that time, as it seems that happens with many elderly with dementia.

As we talked with one of her caregivers, I was hit by another intuitive flash, and found myself telling her another story.

"Mama," I said. "Jolene is here to give you a skin treatment." *Skin treatment*, I asked myself. *Where in the world did that come from?*
"A skin treatment?" she echoed a bit incredulously.
"Yes, they're very special, and so good for you," I replied.

So, I spun the tale. I don't remember now if I invoked the long-dead ghost of Dr. Whorton or not. But whatever was said seemed to do the trick. Mama allowed Jolene to give her a bath.

We never referred to the bath by its proper name again. It was always a skin treatment. She never fought the bath again, but allowed Jolene to bathe her. Only Jolene.

And that was fine with everyone else.

Reflection: Addressing the Intimately Personal Caregiving

Some of the most difficult issues we face in caregiving include incontinence, not bathing, wandering, and problems with elimination. Mother didn't wander, which was a blessing.

If your elderly parent starts to bathe or shower less, or actively resists that well-entrenched ritual, you're not alone. People with dementia will gradually lose their capacity to handle their daily tasks, including self-care. They forget how to bathe and how to dress themselves. Some can actually come to fear water.

Look at eldercare websites and talk with friends and colleagues. Develop a list of tips and strategies that might be helpful in your situation. Every person is different, but there are probably ways that you can approach personal care challenges that make the solution a bit easier, rather than harder.

Often, we can benefit from talking with a professional caregiver, a staff person at a local Senior Center, or someone who has dealt with these specific issues. I believe that good caregivers have developed an amazing set of skills that help them deal successfully with all of these challenges.

Remember that these are challenging situations for everyone. You're looking for progress here. Do the best you can.

Chapter 26: Managing Sundowner's – Her Mother's Summer at Columbia

Mother continued to decline during the almost two years she lived with John in Wyoming. My visits became more frequent because I now lived closer to Mama than I had before. We had excellent caregivers, and John was amazing in the way he managed.

Mama had a wonderful quality of life, almost impossible for most people in such a state of advanced dementia. Almost every day, John or one of the caregivers took her out for a drive. She loved to see the birds, the mountains, and the antelope. She found the wildlife fascinating and looked forward to the drives. They were moments of joy for her.

She continued to play the piano. At this point, she didn't have the skill she'd had in earlier years, but she could still play quite a few tunes, especially "Tea for Two" and other World War II-era songs.

With John's assistance, she was asked once or twice to go to the Senior Center to play. We hoped she would go not only to play, but for socialization and lunch. With our prompting, she reluctantly agreed. She gave her answer in no uncertain terms. "Well, I'll go, but I won't stay. I don't have anything in common with those old folks." She went. She played. She never stayed for lunch. Oh, well. It was a good idea.

Every day near dusk, which was 4 p.m. in the winter in Wyoming, she would begin to become agitated. She would usually be finished with *The Sound of Music* by mid to late afternoon. If she didn't watch it twice, she would look out the window.

We'd have to watch her because she would also often open the door, heating the outdoors and causing the inside temperature to plummet. She would wander back and forth between the living room, dining room, and kitchen. And as the sky became darker, she would usually say: "It's getting late. I have to get back home to Mama."

Gram was born in 1882 and died in 1982, almost twenty years before Mama's Wyoming days. Mother and Dad had taken such good care of Gram at home during her last years. Mother was the baby of the family, and she and Gram were extremely close. She gave Gram nothing but the best, most tender loving care possible.

Mother would keep talking about needing to go, and we would try to distract her or soothe her. But she experienced our efforts as troubling. After all, we were keeping her from getting back to her mother. I remember many times trying to get her to focus on something else, like playing the piano. It didn't work. She could not be distracted. Our efforts to redirect simply made her more anxious and determined.

As the sky would darken, she would become increasingly agitated, begging us to help her get on the road and back home to Birmingham and her mother. It was painful and exhausting. We tried so many things. Nothing seemed to work.

All three of us would talk from time to time about the problem with Sundowner's Syndrome. Most people with Alzheimer's are affected by this syndrome. As the sun begins to set, they become agitated and are often fearful of the darkening world. Turning up the lights helped somewhat, but only as a temporary placating device.

Finally, late one afternoon during one of my visits, she began the litany again about needing to leave, to go home to her mother. I'm not sure where I got the idea, but I said "Mama, don't you remember? Gram isn't home right now. She got an award to study art at Columbia in New York. She's in New York at the Art Institute."

Snap.

"She is?" she said. "Oh, all right." Somehow, I had found the answer that calmed her. Over the rest of that evening and the remainder of my visit, when Mother expressed concerns about needing to go back home to her Mama, I would explain that she was up in New York at Columbia studying art.

It worked. It really worked.

Back in the late 1920s, '30s, and '40s, Gram had been an award-winning Southern artist, well-known for her commissioned portraits of Jefferson Davis and House Speaker Bankhead (father of the famous Tallulah Bankhead). Gram did go to Columbia one summer in the late 1920s to study art. It was a highlight for her and for Mama, and they talked about it with a great deal of fondness. Mother went up to visit her in New York that summer. There are quite a few pictures of them "doing the town," hats and all.

Like so many of the solutions we found for Mama's care, this one came as an intuitive insight, right "out of the blue." These solutions were not rationally deduced at all. Rather, a creative idea would just come to us and we would try it out.

That happened with my response to her when she said to me "You look so familiar," when we were at my Cousin Jenny's house before Tula's memorial service. It was that same intuitive "hit" with *The Sound of Music*. It was that creative brainstorming that convinced us we could move Mama and make it all a story, an adventure.

For much of the remaining year or two of her life, Mother would talk about needing to get back to Birmingham to take care of her mother. We would remind her that Gram was at Columbia studying art. She would nod, remembering that fact. And she would be comforted.

Reflection: Sundowner's and Redirection

Sundowner's Syndrome seems to happen to many people who have Alzheimer's. When the sun starts setting, those with Sundowner's become quite agitated.

There are many excellent resources online that provide us a greater understanding of Sundowner's and tips for how to handle things. In general, caregiving experts encourage us to accept it and learn to navigate the change. In a calm way, we can redirect our loved one. Whenever possible, engage them in an activity they enjoy.

Provide loving attention, reminding them that you are there for them, you care for them, and they will be all right.

Redirecting often works well, especially when you refocus them on an activity they enjoy.

Seek guidance and support from local caregivers, your family and friends, and your loved one's healthcare provider.

Try different things and be creative, as people have different ways that Sundowner's affects them, and different ways they can be redirected. Go with the flow and help them to solve what are usually their imaginary problems.

Chapter 27: Taking Time and Living in the Now

Caring for Mama during her final years with Alzheimer's taught me the importance of living in the now. Time was a shape-shifting enemy for all of us. We never knew what a new day would bring. Over the years, we changed our expectations countless times.

It was no longer important to have reality-based conversations. We just talked about whatever interested her in the moment. Sometimes our conversations would go something like this:

"Oh, Mama. See the bird?"
"Where?"
"Over there. In the tree."
"Pretty. I like the birds."
"Hear the birds. They are singing."
"Yes, singing birds."

"Look, there goes a car."
"Isn't that a big car?"
"That car's too big."
"I know, I wouldn't want to drive a car that big."
"I like our car."

We would talk that way about almost everything during the last nine months or so of her life. It kept her connected with us and grounded us.

By this time, Mother had lost a good bit of her vocabulary. Thank goodness she had a very large one to begin with. Building your vocabulary has a new level of importance for me now. She had a lot to start with, which enabled her to cope a lot longer than most.

A large vocabulary full of synonyms served as one of her best tools in the fight against the progression of dementia. That, and her music.

We would watch *The Sound of Music* together. Once or twice a day.

We would go for rides.

I would play the piano. And she would play the piano. Although her repertoire diminished substantially, she could still play a few pieces until a few months before she died.

We would listen to music, and John would often play the piano for us. He composed music for piano. It was always a treat to hear him play something new he had just finished.

Her favorite foods became a much bigger deal, and we would "ooh" and "aah" over candy, cookies, and ice cream.

We would read selections from some of her favorite authors, focusing on old, well-loved, and well-known writings. Mama had been an English major and loved Shakespeare. We would read from some of the bard's best-known dialogues. She enjoyed a popular news anchor who wrote a book about traveling through the US, and John read sections of that book to her for many months. We read the 23rd Psalm. We said the Lord's Pray at night.

Sometimes, we would just sit.

Reflection: Connecting Without Many Words

Spending time with a loved one doing simple things is a blessing, and it was one of the gifts of Mother's Alzheimer's. We were forced to focus on the basics, the simplest things. Our language became simpler as we looked for ways to reflect on and talk about a shared experience. Those simple conversations helped her stay more engaged and energized her.

It was helpful to just sit with Mama.

We live in a society in the US that values talk and action. We also have a growing trend focused on spirituality, mindfulness, and living in the present. It can be very helpful to everyone involved to spend time just sitting together. You might just sit, revel in nature, read, or work on a report.

Or just sit.

Being present with someone during the last part of their life provides a gift to both.

Chapter 28: Thanksgiving, My Last Visit with Mama

My last, and one of my nicest visits with Mama, was Thanksgiving of 2002. By this time, she was talking very little. She had lost some more weight and was quite frail.

I had decided that I would spend close to a week visiting. I had been quite a workaholic during my younger and middle adult years, and I was in a period where I was taking baby steps to develop a more balanced life. I am so glad I took that extra time.

What stands out for me as I remember that visit was how calm and peaceful we both were. It was just a nice time all around. It was pleasant and easy. That, in our family, is a major accomplishment.

She and I spent a lot of time together, just sitting and talking about little things. We watched *The Sound of Music* together.

We went on a lot of rides through the Wyoming countryside, counting cattle, deer, and antelope. Sometimes we would start singing about how the deer and the antelope play when we saw them.

And we just sat. Companionably, often in silence or with limited conversation.

It was a pleasant and unhurried time.

I realized that she was very frail and would probably not last much longer. I just didn't realize that it would happen so quickly.

Reflection: Discovering the Goodbyes

By this time, Mama was extremely frail. In spite of the many supercharged high-calorie, high-protein shakes we made for her, she consumed little, and her weight had dropped to just over ninety pounds.

Her vocabulary had shrunk even more than her body. The once articulate and well-read master of the right phrase could only utter a few comments. Her brain was full of the deadly plaque that was slowly choking it off through its maddening proliferation, like the Alabama kudzu.

When people talk about the impact of Alzheimer's, they usually mention two things:

1. *The disease robs people of their very essence. It takes their brains, and their ability to think, communicate, and act.*
2. *Even when they are severely impaired, a spark remains and we can still connect in some way.*

Both are true.

If you're able to somehow live in the dynamic tension created by that paradox, you're living in sacred space. You and your loved one will benefit from the process of living with those two realities.

Chapter 29: Her Last Day – Debussy, Our Goodbyes and the 23rd Psalm

Like most caregivers, I was juggling too much, overly stressed, and not taking enough time for rest. Pushing myself to finish work deadlines before returning to Wyoming, I was driving back to Santa Fe from a long day of meetings out of town when stress caught up with me. Driving tired and distracted, I had a car accident that was serious enough to total my car.

After the officer on site took my information, I called John to let him know what happened. John responded with the strangest comments:

"I'm so glad you called," he said.
"Why?"
"Because Mother has been agitated and upset for the last half hour or so. She's been asking about you, saying 'what's wrong with Anne Hays?'"
"What?"
"Yes, she's been very upset. She's been pacing, asking about you. Worried that something bad had happened."

As I talked with them both, I realized that Mama was more present, articulate, and connected than I had heard her in a good while. I reassured them that I was all right, but shaken.

The police officer on the scene was wonderful, and he offered to take me to a hotel after we finished the paperwork.

Later, both John and I talked. We agreed the incident was strange and seemed full of coincidence. Or God's sticky fingers were all over it. The experience seemed to me to represent something more than a synchronicity. Mama was connected at an energetic or ethereal level and she got upset at the same time of my accident and repeatedly asked if I was all right.

I've believed for a long time that the veil between this world and the next can often be quite thin. I've also believed that there are many different ways of knowing. Somehow, both seemed to have been present in that situation. I can't figure it out and don't try. There had been an incredibly powerful connection, which has meant a great deal to me in the years since.

The next week, and the last week before my return to Wyoming, my "To Do" list had grown to include finding a new car. During the beginning of the second week of December, John and I talked daily, sometimes a few times a day. Mother had caught a cold and was not feeling well. We were both worried.

When I talked with Mother on the phone, she sounded chipper but tired and frail. I had planned to drive back up to Wyoming in mid-December, after winding up some meetings scheduled on a new project. John felt that Mother might be slipping, but neither of us thought she would decline as quickly as she did.

A few days before I was scheduled to go to Wyoming, John and I had a long talk about Mother's condition. He reported that she had been feeling sicker, that caregivers were spending additional time with her, and the Visiting Nurse Service nurse was coming more often. I offered to come up earlier and reschedule the meetings, but after further discussion we both felt that it would be fine for me to drive up on the 17th.

Sometime earlier in the day the 17th, John told me that Mother's breathing had become labored, and that he and Dottie from Visiting Nurse Services asked her if she wanted to go to the hospital. She said "no." Dottie had discussed the pros and cons of putting Mother on oxygen, as her blood oxygen levels were beginning to decline.

John talked with Tom and me about this. We all agreed that the oxygen would simply prolong the inevitable, and that Mother would probably be frightened of the tubes. It was one of the toughest decisions we ever made. We also knew that it was exactly the decision Mother would have made for herself. I gained a newfound appreciation of Mother's standoff with the young doctor when Gram was dying.

We did decide to enroll Mother in hospice care, which turned out to last for little over a day. The caregivers and nurse who had been with her for so long were the real anchors for her and for us.

I worked to wrap up, and headed north straight from my meetings in Taos, through the mountains. By the time I was entering Colorado, a snowstorm had started. By the time I was close to Denver, the slopes had iced and traffic was at a near standstill.

The Colorado crews were finally able to clear the roads. Driving past Denver, I realized that I would probably be able to make Buffalo that night, just very late. During the late afternoon and evening, I had been talking with John and Mother.

When I stopped for gas in Cheyenne, I called again and had what was to be my last conversation with Mama. I reassured her once again that I was on my way.

"Mama, I'm almost there. I'll be there soon. I love you."
"I love you, too," she said.

I drove as fast as I could, but missed her last moments by just a few hours. Initially, I was devastated. But as I lived with the loss, I realized that we had said goodbye in a sense at Thanksgiving, with that peace-filled, joyful few days of being together. John allowed her to slip away naturally, without any extraordinary measures, as she wanted.

John is one of those rare people with a stratospherically high IQ and a limitlessly compassionate heart. His care for Mother during her last few days was a testament to both.

Knowing her wishes, he gathered the caregiving resources to surround her in the ways she wanted. When Mama was no longer able to get out of bed, a day or so before her death, he had the piano moved into her room so that she could hear him playing.

Throughout the last day, he would play Mozart, Bach, Ravel, and Debussy. He made sure that she was supported in her journey by her familiar favorites, like Bach's *Sheep May Safely Graze*, and Debussy's *Girl with The Flaxen Hair*, as well as some of her most loved hymns. He read the 23rd Psalm.

John told me that about a half hour after my call to them from Cheyenne, Mother slipped out of consciousness. Her breathing slowed and became shallower. Betsy Blue Eyes, one of her cats, came to lie beside her head as she was slipping away.

Tom and Ann came out to join us a day or two later, and the four of us made funeral plans. They were rather complex and included a service in Wyoming, a burial in the family plot in Birmingham, and a memorial in Winston-Salem where Mother and Dad had lived for over thirty years.

For quite some time, we second-guessed our decisions. Should she have gone to the hospital? Was it appropriate to defer the oxygen? Should I have canceled my meetings and left earlier?

Over time, we realized that each of us did the best we could, given the conditions of the day. We worked together as a team, and made decisions jointly, which was amazing and very much unlike our often-dysfunctional family dynamic. We consulted one another. We were committed to doing what we thought Mother wanted, and what was best for her.

There is a great deal we learned from the experience. As we were making plans for her funeral and memorial service, we began to reflect on our journey together.

Reflecting on the Experience

All four of us reflected on Mama's last weeks and months for some time. It had been a long journey. We were exhausted. We were also sad at her decline, and sad to see her go.

What helped was time to reflect about it in the months after her passing. It also helped to talk with each other about things.

I was so sad that I missed her passing by just a few hours, and wondered why I had not left earlier. I was hard on myself. All of us were second-thinking decisions in the aftermath.

We were comforted by friends and family who came to her service in Buffalo, and those who came to the memorial in Winston-Salem. There were not many people at her burial in Birmingham; however, people from the Red Cross came and brought a Red Cross flag. That was so moving.

After some time, I realized that all of us had done a really good job at taking care of her and her assets in the way she would have wanted. We did the best we could.

Finally, I realized that we did all that we could, and that was enough.

That's grace whispering.

Resources for Caregiving

The following provides a list of helpful resources for you as you look at providing care to your parent, spouse, or other loved one. These core community resources are described based on the category or type of service. National and international resources are listed at the end of the article.

Sometimes it is difficult to identify needed community resources to help with an elderly person's care. Professionals in this and related fields often find that caregiving resources grow and change quickly, and it can be difficult to keep up with these changes. Family members are even more confused as they try to discover and then access appropriate resources. Some of the confusion can be allayed if family members utilize this list and work with their local Senior Center or other aging resources to help map out those resources that are most needed and available.

I. Resources in the US

A. Older Adult Services: The Big Picture

The "backbone" of community services for the elderly has been the Administration on Aging funded federal Title XX services for older adults authorized by the Older Americans Act. The Older Americans Act was initially passed in 1965, and reauthorized most recently in 2011. It establishes the federal Administration on Aging to oversee and fund older adult services. The law provides the policies, defines the services, and describes the funding parameters for services for older adults.

In 1973–1974, the federal Administration on Aging established Area Agencies on Aging and funding for social services for older adults through the states. In the early 1980s, the Administration on Aging was involved in nursing home reform through an omnibus reconciliation act. Later, it dealt with the growing demand for and regulation of caregivers, discrimination against the elderly and elder rights.

The federal Administration for Community Living, which manages these programs, states that the Older Americans Act (OAA):

> *... is considered to be a major vehicle for the organization and delivery of social and nutrition services to this group and their caregivers. It authorizes a wide array of service programs through a national network of 56 state agencies on aging, 618 area agencies on aging, nearly 20,000 service providers, 281 Tribal organizations, and 1 Native Hawaiian organization representing 400 Tribes. The OAA also includes community Service employment for low-income older Americans; training, research, and demonstration activities in the field of aging; and vulnerable elder rights protection activities.*

Find out more information about the Older Americans Act and its services by searching acl.gov and "Older Americans Act."

B. Core State and Community Resources

Core social service, nutrition, transportation, and home care programs at the community level are often funded through Administration on Aging grants to the states. Many of these services are offered through a county or local city Senior Center or local/regional Area Agency on Aging. Senior Centers are often nonprofit agencies; however, some centers are run by local government entities. In larger communities, one can find a good number of Title XX funded organization.

For more information about Title XX funded services, contact the Administration on Aging's website by typing in those words, and/or contact your state's Agency on Aging.

C. Other Community Resources

There are a number of services in many local communities. The larger the community, the greater and more diverse the programs and services. The following represent some of the most frequently found local resources.

Senior Centers. These provide a range of services to older adults, usually age sixty and older. The larger centers have multiple streams of funding. They often provide a range of social, educational, and fitness activities; lunch and nutrition services; transportation, and often some level of visiting and/or home care services. Many centers that are nonprofits receive additional funding from grants, contracts, and donors, which allows them to further develop and expand services beyond core services funded by the Agency on Aging. Some have also built out services that can be funded by Medicare and Medicaid.

Adult Day Center. They represent adult day care services, usually in a center-based facility, to frail elderly who are not safe staying at home alone without a caregiver. These are especially helpful for adult children who live in the same home and work outside the home during the day. This enables people to keep frail elders in the family setting while retaining their jobs. Many services are covered through grant funding or Medicaid, with some services that may be covered through Medicare.

Visiting Nurse Services (VNS). Located in most major metropolitan areas, Visiting Nurse Services is a nonprofit home health care agency founded almost 100 years ago. It provides home health care and hospice services in many communities. Services to older adults comprise a large portion of many local VNS agencies. VNS home care services allow many older adults to remain in their homes by providing assistance to help people with basic activities of daily living (ADLs).

Meals on Wheels. Local Meals on Wheels programs provide home-delivered meals to homebound people five days a week. Services to older adults represent a significant part of home-delivered meals.

Local Hospice Organizations. Many communities have a freestanding local hospice nonprofit agency or a hospice program related to a local hospital or other large organization. Large metro areas may have multiple hospice programs. Hospice care is a critically needed part of the service mix, and a growing need. If your loved one is moving toward palliative care, hospice resources can be extremely helpful. Many provide care to your loved one in their own home; some have hospice facilities. Most also provide supports to family caregivers.

Caregiving. Nonprofits and businesses provide a range of caregiving services. Some of the strongest in the field have excellent quality records. Check thoroughly, as there are often significant differences among local providers with respect to the quality of care provided as well as costs.

Counseling. Therapeutic services are available in many different settings. We have a growing group of therapists, counselors, and case managers with expertise in family counseling as well as working with adult children of frail elderly. Look for this expertise.

Legal Issues. These often include developing financial and health care Power of Attorney or general Power of Attorney. Other issues can include developing wills and trusts, identifying affairs that need to be handled by the adult children, and, in some cases guardianship. In some communities, there are Senior Citizens' Law resources that provide pro bono and/or sliding fee scale services. Find attorneys with expertise in elder law.

Financial Issues. In addition to issues mentioned above, many families find that the costs for elder care to be excessive, sometimes stripping family resources. Resources can include nonprofit sliding fee scale services, dual eligible Medicare/Medicaid coverage, and county health care funds in many states.

D. National Online Resources

The following include a list of some of the most popular and helpful national resources, updated from time to time as needed.

Administration on Aging. The federal Administration on Aging (AOA) provides funding and resources to all US states and territories for a range of programs for older adults. States provide funding for a number of important community-based programs, to include local Senior Centers. In many communities, funding also covers some level of home care, transportation, and respite care. The AOA has extensive website resources, and is recommended as a "first stop" in your research. Check your state Agency on Aging website for more information about local community resources.

Alzheimer's Association. The Alzheimer's Association has been a major resource in the field of aging for decades, and provides excellent resources about the disease. It offers practical information and guidance to help caregivers to cope with the impact of Alzheimer's on families. Also provides contacts for local chapters and community resources.

AARP - American Association of Retired Persons. AARP is one of the largest associations in the US, with a membership base in the tens of millions. They provide information, resources, and referrals on many topics of concern to older adults and their families.

Benefits Check Up. Benefits Check Up is a comprehensive website of the National Council on Aging that provides information about benefits that may be available to you or your loved one. It's a simple way to discover what may be available for you.

Healthfinder. Site hosted by the federal government's Department of Health and Human Services. Provides health information and resources.

Medicare (Centers for Medicare and Medicaid). Important federal government resource describing the Medicare program, types of plans and policies, and covered conditions. Also includes information about fraud and links to other helpful government publications. Website lists state and local community resources, and information about nearby local government offices that can help.

National Alliance for Caregiving (NAC). NAC is a nonprofit coalition of national organizations focusing on issues of family caregiving. Alliance members include grassroots organizations, professional associations, service organizations, disease-specific organizations, a government agency, and corporations. NAC has a great deal of information on its website, including research findings, resources for caregivers, and information about state and local coalitions. It also provides updates about important legislation.

National Clearinghouse for Long Term Care Information. This US Department of Health and Human Services website provides information and resources to help families plan for future long-term care (LTC) needs. The site provides information about long-term care, how to pay for services, resources and links to state and local community resources.

National Family Caregivers Association (NFCA). NFCA provides support, resources and advocacy to the more than 65 million Americans who care for loved ones with a chronic illness, disability or the frailties of old age. The website provides resources and information and has a program to connect caregivers. It also provides information about advocacy and legislative issues.

II. International Resources

There are a number of helpful international resources for Alzheimer's, dementia, caregiving and elder care. Many of these include resources for different countries. It is recommended that you research aging resources in your own country by searching for national governmental resources, as well as NGOs working in the field; studies and resources for your country or region; and aging resources for your community. The following may provide a broad overview.

Alzheimer's Disease International. This represents one of the leading international organizations working in the area of Alzheimer's.

World Economic Forum. An invitation-only network of economic, governmental, social, healthcare, and philanthropic world leaders. One of its recent articles is "Elderly Care: How can Countries Cope with Ageing Populations?"

Aging Alone: Elder Care Infrastructure in the EU. Report indicates most European Countries provide more elder care, enshrined in social rights policies.

European Social Network (ESN), a working group on ageing and social care, with a focus on integrating healthcare and social care services.

European Aging Network (EAN), includes more than 10,000 aging care providers from across the European continent.

Ageing International. Publication for international scholars and researchers.

GlobalAgeing. Global Aging Network

National Institute on Aging's HRS International Family of Studies. NIA's Health and Retirement (HRS) Studies include research on aging in many countries.

United Nations. Research and reports on elder care in different countries. Including article "Caregiving in an Ageing World."

ABOUT THE AUTHOR

Rev. Dr. Anne Hays Egan is an organizational development consultant based near Santa Fe, NM. She has worked extensively with local, regional, and state community building initiatives. The author has extensive expertise with aging, health, and behavioral health research, community needs assessments, planning, service coordination, and system development work. She has helped agencies to plan and fund service networks, including services to older adults.

She is also known as a researcher and writer in the field, with over 50 publications to her credit. She has published widely on topics related to aging, health, behavioral health, nonprofit organizations, public policy, and building effective programs and services.

She was the publisher of *The Digest of Nonprofit Management*, the first national newsletter on nonprofit management, which was sold to The Taft Group.

Anne lived in shared housing with Maggie Kuhn, the founder of the Gray Panthers, who was one of her models and mentors. She is a retired Presbyterian minister and partially retired system development and community building consultant. Anne loves to travel and plays violin with the Santa Fe Community Orchestra and quartets.

Anne's other books include *Building Communities of Hope*, and two upcoming books. These are *Raising Hell for the Greater Good* and *God's Eyes*. Watch for new books that will come out at the end of 2023 and in 2024.

Made in the USA
Columbia, SC
03 January 2024